chocolate-covered katie

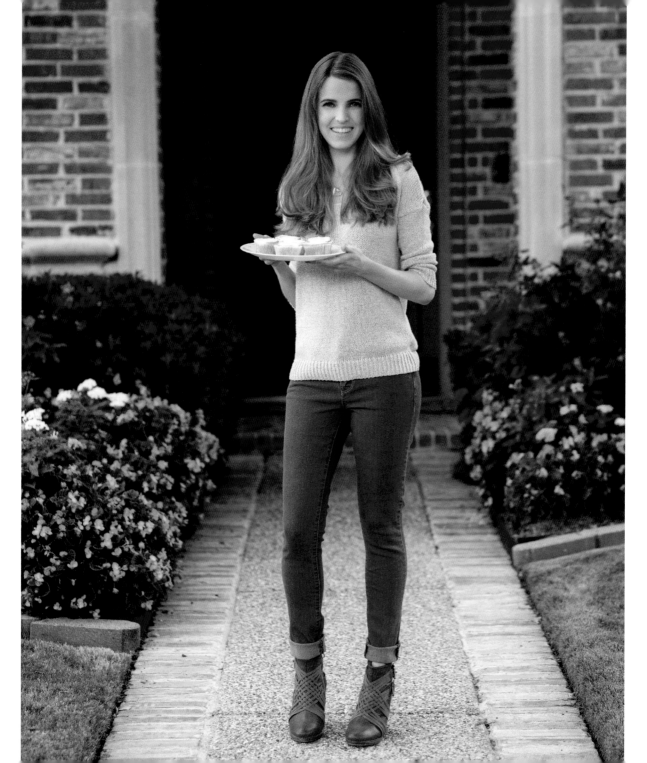

chocolate-covered katie

over 80 delicious
recipes that are
secretly GOOD for you

Katie Higgins

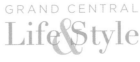

GRAND CENTRAL
Life&Style

New York Boston

Grand Central Life & Style
Hachette Book Group
1290 Avenue of the Americas
New York, NY 10104

www.GrandCentralLifeandStyle.com

Printed in the United States of America

Design by Amy Sly

Q-MA

First Edition: January 2015
10 9 8 7 6 5 4

Grand Central Life & Style is an imprint of Grand Central Publishing.

The Grand Central Life & Style name and logo are trademarks of Hachette Book Group, Inc.

The Hachette Speakers Bureau provides a wide range of authors for speaking events. To find out more, go to www.HachetteSpeakersBureau.com or call (866) 376-6591.

The publisher is not responsible for websites (or their content) that are not owned by the publisher.

Library of Congress Cataloging-in-Publication Data
Higgins, Katie.

Chocolate-covered Katie : over 80 delicious recipes that are secretly good for you / Katie Higgins.—First edition.

    pages cm

  Includes index.

  ISBN 978-1-4555-9970-7 (trade pbk.)—ISBN 978-1-4555-9969-1 (ebook) 1. Chocolate desserts. 2. Cooking (Chocolate). I. Title.

  TX773.H47 2015

  641.6'374—dc23

                                           2014017846

This cookbook is dedicated to every single person who has ever visited my website, chocolatecoveredkatie.com. When I started the blog, I didn't believe anyone would actually read it, and I appreciate you all more than you will ever know!

The book is also dedicated to my mother, a woman who exemplifies the most courage, compassion, and selflessness of anyone I've ever met. Her unwavering support and encouragement give me the confidence to reach for my dreams, chocolate-covered spatula in hand.

acknowledgments

So many people have made this book possible, and I am incredibly grateful to each one of you.

Thank you, first, to my parents and grandparents for instilling in me a culinary passion and for teaching me early on the importance of food in a social setting. Parties just would not have been the same without Mimi's macaroni or Grandma's stuffed cabbage.

To my sister, my cooking, baking, and potion-making partner in crime, who always let me have the bigger half whenever chocolate was involved. I love you so much and am proud to be your sister (even if it did take years of biting you and pulling your hair to realize this).

To Sara Weiss, my editor at Grand Central Publishing, who patiently guided me through the process of writing my first book. You were a complete joy to work with, and I found myself constantly marveling at your incredible work ethic (hour-long phone conversations when I needed reassurance, responding to e-mails at 9 p.m. on a Saturday, the list goes on and on…). I cannot say enough good things about you.

To the talented Lara Ferroni and Sara Kiesling for making this book beautiful. I hadn't met Sara Kiesling before she arrived at my home one day to take author photos. But seven hours—and many animated conversations—later, she left as one of my dear friends.

To Lisa Grubka at Fletcher and Co., and to Amanda Englander, who envisioned this cookbook before I did and talked me into writing it. Thank you for believing in me.

To Amy Sly, the book's designer, for lending your artistic eye to the project, and to Deri Reed, and Siri Silleck at Grand Central Publishing, for helping me through the long editing process.

To my recipe testers and friends, for giving me your honest opinions and for helping me to eat batch after batch after batch of brownies and cookies!

And finally, to everyone who picked up a copy of this book. Thank you for making my dreams come true.

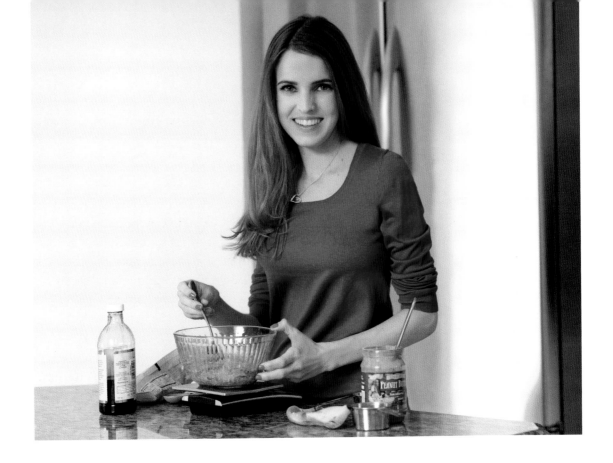

author's note

All of the recipes in this book come with a nutritional analysis located at the bottom of the page. Nutritional analyses are meant to serve as general guidelines, and, due to ingredient and brand variations, may not completely reflect the specific ingredients you are using. Analyses have been calculated with spelt flour whenever it is listed as an option and Silk almond milk when "milk of choice" is called for. Optional ingredients or crusts are not included in calculations, and when more than one option for an ingredient is listed, nutrition facts are based on the lowest calorie option. When a serving range is given, nutrition facts are based on the smallest serving size.

contents

introduction 10

1 the chocolate-covered kitchen 13

2 cookies, brownies & bars 23

3 dessert for breakfast 63

4 ice cream, milkshakes & smoothies 103

5 pies, cakes & cupcakes 137

6 puddings, dips, frostings & more 175

stevia conversion chart 200
metric conversion charts 201
index 202

chocolate-covered katie

this is not
your average
cookbook.

Many diet books on the market today will tell you that in order to lose weight or get healthier, you need to cut back on the sweets. But when you forbid yourself your favorite foods, what happens? You end up craving those treats even more! Denying yourself what you desire most can be a recipe for disaster, often resulting in massive sugar binges that leave you feeling guilty and dangerously out of control.

Instead, why not do your body a favor and honor your true cravings? With this cookbook, you need never skip dessert again. You'll learn easy ways to say YES to cinnamon rolls, milkshakes, and chocolate cream pie while still fitting into your skinny jeans, feeling great, and achieving the best, most-vibrant health of your life.

Six years ago, frustrated with what was passing for good healthy desserts, I started a small food blog called *Chocolate-Covered Katie* (chocolatecoveredkatie.com). Using only real ingredients—no artificial sweeteners, no fake "diet" foods—my goal was to prove that healthy desserts can taste just as rich and luxurious as their fat-and-sugar-laden counterparts...and sometimes even better!

I've always been passionate about dessert. While classmates cited popcorn and pizza among their favorite foods, my own young life revolved around brownies, cookies, and hot fudge sundaes. It wasn't uncommon for me to buy *two* Snickers bars at the movies, or dive headfirst into a giant piece of chocolate cake for breakfast.

Eventually, however, the massive quantities of fat and sugar in these beloved chocolate

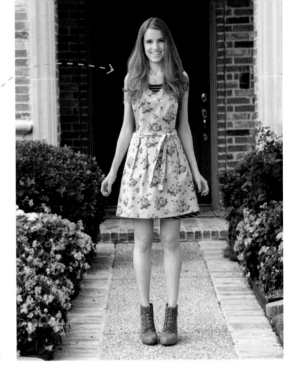

treats began to leave me feeling completely drained of energy, and during my freshman year of college it finally went too far. With bed, books, and food crammed into a tiny dorm room, chocolate was never more than an arm's-reach away, and I took full advantage. I kept the mini fridge stocked with cakes from my favorite bakery (conveniently located just miles from campus) and would often eat multiple slices by nightfall. I was constantly tired and experienced "sugar high" headaches at least once a week. Something needed to change.

Around this same time, many of my friends were waging wars of their own against dessert and its famous accompanying consequence: the freshman 15. Feeling unhealthy and unhappy, we decided to put up a collective fight, banning Ben & Jerry's from the premises and replacing candy bars with carrot sticks and 100-calorie packs. We searched online for "healthy dessert" recipes, but every

single one we tried fell flat. Those fat-free bean brownies? Yes, they tasted as terrible as they sounded. My friends attempted to put on brave faces. "They're okay…for a healthy dessert," they'd say with a shrug.

But I didn't want something that tasted good just for a healthy dessert. I wanted dessert to taste good, period.

Chocolate-Covered Katie offers just that. Each of the desserts in this book gets the stamp of approval from healthy eaters and junk-food eaters alike. Here, you will find over 80 healthier versions of your favorite treats, from classic chocolate chip cookies to New York–style cheesecake, so smooth and creamy that you'll be dreaming about it for months.

So what makes these recipes a better choice than traditional desserts? Many are much lower in sugar, are 100 percent whole grain, and offer important vitamins and nutrients such as dietary fiber, potassium, and essential omega-3s. I've even snuck vegetables into some of the recipes. But I promise you, no one will ever be able to tell!

All of the recipes in the book are free of refined carbohydrates, provided the option for whole grain flour is used. They have the option of being completely free of refined sugar as well, and all are free of trans fats. Only heart-healthy fats are used.

The ingredients called for in the recipes have no harmful chemicals, additives, or unhealthy food dyes often found in packaged sweets. Each recipe is 100 percent cholesterol-free, provided you use non-dairy ingredients when given the option.

Thanks to their high-quality and nutritious ingredients, many of these recipes are not only healthier than their traditional counterparts; they are downright *good for you*!

Studies have proven that eating chocolate—especially dark chocolate—in moderation is actually beneficial for your health. In one such study, researchers followed 1,000 volunteers and found that the participants who regularly ate dark chocolate more than twice a week weighed *less* than those who did not indulge as frequently![*]

The antioxidant flavonols in dark chocolate have been shown to help lower cholesterol, increase blood flow to the brain, lower insulin levels, decrease appetite, and even increase happiness.[†]

Please note, of course, that the information above does not mean you should eat dessert with reckless abandon; but the same can be said about any food. Did you know that too much broccoli can cause acid poisoning, and that too much raw kale can inhibit thyroid function? It's true! Moderation is key.

You can eat the desserts in this cookbook every day as part of a healthy diet, but do remember to include lots of fruits and vegetables in your non-dessert meals. The American Heart Association recommends eating eight or more daily servings of fruits and vegetables. Luckily for you, many of the recipes in this book can count toward that total! Never again will you be forced to choose between good health and good taste. You can have your cake (preferably *chocolate* cake!) and eat it too.

---

[*] http://archinte.jamanetwork.com/article.aspx?articleid=1108800

[†] http://www.huffingtonpost.com/2013/11/07/chocolate-health-benefits_n_4214777.html

1

the chocolate-covered kitchen

With just a few steps, you'll be ready to turn your own kitchen into a chocolate-covered oasis. Here's an overview of the tools, ingredients, tips, and tricks that might prove helpful along the way.

tools of the trade

Good news: Many of the kitchen tools used to make the desserts in this cookbook might already be in your pantry! You also don't need to buy every item listed here—it is simply a list of the tools mentioned in the book.

food processor

If your budget allows room for only one cooking gadget, a food processor is the way to go. A blender can get the job done in many cases, but there are some instances in which a blender just won't cut it (pun intended). For example, in my bean-based recipes, a food processor is necessary to achieve that smooth "cookie dough" texture. I've noted where a food processor is required, but otherwise feel free to use either a blender or a food processor. In terms of brand, I am partial to Cuisinart. My own 7-cup machine is almost 15 years old and has processed thousands of recipes. Talk about $200 well spent!

magic bullet blender

This miniature blender is great for smaller-serving recipes, such as smoothies and frostings. It's not incredibly expensive and can go in the dishwasher, making cleanup a breeze. However, you can easily make every single one of the recipes in this book without a Magic Bullet.

vitamix blender

Known as a high-speed blender, this extremely powerful machine is like the superhero of the blending world. It turns nuts, seeds, frozen fruit, and other hard-to-blend items into smooth purees in seconds. Owning a Vitamix can be a great investment if you're the type who makes your own soups, nut butters, and ice creams. My favorite thing to make in the Vitamix is homemade ice cream (such as the recipes starting on page 104). However, owning this machine is not an absolute requirement for any of the recipes in this book.

measuring spoons

Look for a set that includes a $1/8$-teaspoon spoon. If you can find a set—either in a kitchen store or online—that includes a $1/16$-teaspoon spoon, that's even better! If not, just fill up your $1/8$ teaspoon halfway when a recipe calls for $1/16$ teaspoon of an ingredient. Precision can make a world of difference to the final taste of a recipe, especially when it comes to concentrated ingredients such as salt or pure stevia extract.

food scale

If you are serious about baking and want the most consistent results possible, the best thing you can do is invest as little as $20 in a food scale. Measuring cups vary depending on the manufacturer and how tightly you pack something, but grams are always exact. (For a cup-to-gram chart, see page 201.) Plus, this way there is no need to worry about scraping peanut butter or sticky sweetener out of a measuring cup…just put the mixing bowl on the food scale and measure straight into it. Saves on cleanup, too!

baking pans

Some of the specific baking pans called for in these recipes include an 8-inch round pan, an 8-inch square pan, a 9x13-inch rectangular pan, an 8½-inch springform pan, a 10-inch springform pan, a 12-cup muffin tin, and a 12-cup or 24-cup mini muffin tin. If you don't have a mini muffin tin, no problem! A regular muffin tin will suffice.

odds 'n' ends

Besides those listed above, a few other supplies you might want to have on hand are: parchment paper, baking sheets, gallon-sized resealable plastic bags, mixing bowls, cupcake liners, and a spatula.

what's in the cupboard

Below is a list of ingredients that are commonly used throughout this book. You might already own a lot of them!

sweeteners

For the best taste and texture, my recipes will often call for more than one type of sweetener. And while it's a good rule of thumb that any sweetener—no matter the type—be used in moderation, some options are healthier than others. Below is a bit more about the various natural sweeteners you will find in this book:

Blackstrap molasses: A surprisingly nutritious sweetener produced by boiling sugarcane juice. The thick syrup is high in iron and calcium, with a gingerbread flavor. Look for it in the baking aisle of health food stores or in some mainstream grocery stores. Regular molasses can always be substituted without compromising flavor, although it has fewer health benefits.

Coconut sugar: This sugar comes from the coconut palm tree, as opposed to sugarcane. It falls much lower on the glycemic index than white sugar, meaning your blood sugar won't spike as quickly as it would with regular sugar. Coconut sugar is high in potassium, zinc, and iron. It can be subbed in a 1-to-1 ratio for white sugar in any of the recipes.

Dates: Many of the recipes in this book rely on dried dates—high in fiber and potassium—to add delicious sweetness without any refined sugar. Look for whole, pitted dates near where raisins are sold in most mainstream grocery stores. I like to use Sun-Maid dates, which I find to be softer (and less expensive) than Medjool dates.

Raw agave: Agave is an unrefined liquid sweetener made from the sap of the agave plant. Proponents of agave appreciate its low-glycemic index (valuable for diabetics), while naysayers point out its high fructose content, which some studies have linked to increased cravings and possible weight gain. Currently the evidence is inconclusive. Superfood or super evil? I treat agave like any other sugar—best used in moderation. If you'd prefer not to use it, other options are listed in the recipes.

Stevia: An all-natural herb that is up to 300 times sweeter than sugar, pure stevia has no calories, no carbohydrates, and no effect on blood glucose. I often use stevia in my recipes as a way to cut back on sugar while still maintaining optimum sweetness. I exclusively use NuNaturals stevia, as it is the only brand I've found to not have a bitter aftertaste. For more on stevia and how to use it, see the Stevia Conversion Chart on page 200.

Sucanat: A contraction of Sugar Cane Natural, Sucanat is simply sugar that has not been bleached and stripped of all its nutrients. It lends a delightful molasses-like flavor to recipes.

Xylitol: A non-artificial, diabetic-friendly sweetener found in the fibers of many fruits and vegetables, xylitol has fewer calories than sugar and is absorbed more slowly into the bloodstream. It has also been shown to improve dental health. Xylitol has no known toxicity in humans, although some people may experience a laxative effect from excessive consumption. (Do not feed xylitol to dogs.) This sweetener can be used interchangeably with white sugar in most recipes. An exception to this rule is in recipes that call for yeast, as the xylitol will inhibit rising.

flours

Once you venture outside the realm of plain white flour, you'll discover a whole new world of possibilities: Spelt flour! Oat flour! Coconut flour! Each whole grain flour has its own unique flavor and texture profile, and trying out a new flour in an old recipe might just lead you to a result you like even better than the original! Below is a bit more about the various flour options you will find in this book:

Coconut flour: Available in health food stores, online, and even in many mainstream grocery stores, coconut flour gives baked goods a rich and buttery taste. It's extremely high in fiber, with 12 grams per $\frac{1}{4}$ cup! (As a comparison, the same amount of all-purpose flour has just 1 gram of fiber.) Coconut flour soaks up water like a sponge and in most cases *cannot* be equally subbed for other flours in a given recipe.

Oat flour: A slightly sweet flour made from finely ground oats. In fact, you can even make this whole grain flour at home by simply putting rolled oats in a food processor or coffee grinder and grinding until a fine flour consistency is achieved. In baked goods, it is best not to substitute oat flour for all of the wheat flour, as it may yield a gummy result. For gluten-free bakers, be sure to look for certified-gluten-free oats or oat flour.

Whole grain spelt flour: My go-to flour for baking, this flour offers health benefits similar to those of traditional whole wheat flour (whole grains and lots of dietary fiber) but results in desserts that are much lighter and fluffier.

Whole wheat pastry flour: A whole grain flour with a lighter texture than regular whole wheat flour, this is my second favorite flour choice behind spelt flour. It can often be substituted in an equal amount for spelt flour, although I have not personally tried it in any of the recipes where it isn't specifically mentioned as an option.

Bob's Red Mill gluten-free all-purpose baking flour: This wheat-free flour is a combination of garbanzo flour, potato starch, tapioca flour, sorghum flour, and fava bean flour, and it is safe for those with celiac disease or a sensitivity to wheat or gluten. You will see it as an option in many of my baked-goods recipes. You are welcome to substitute a different brand of gluten-free flour in the recipes as long as you are okay with the possibility that it might not turn out well.

All-purpose flour: This is your basic "white" flour. It has been stripped of most of its vitamins, minerals, and fiber, and it does not qualify as a whole grain flour. However, you will see all-purpose flour listed as an option in some of the recipes, as I know whole grain flour is not always available depending on where you live. Or, perhaps you're not ready to completely change the way you cook. If this is the case, making these recipes with white flour is a good compromise or starting point: While using the refined flour might make your dessert less healthy, it will still be health*ier* (i.e., lower in sugar, calories, and unhealthy fats and chemicals) than the traditional recipe.

fats

For years, people believed all fat was bad. However, extensive research now proves there are some types of fats that, when eaten in moderation, are not only good for you, but are absolutely essential for a healthy diet. These so-called "good fats" can lower your cholesterol, improve your skin, hair, and nails, and reduce your risk of stroke and heart disease. Below is a bit more about the various healthy fats included in the recipes in this book:

Coconut butter: Not to be confused with coconut oil (think peanut butter and peanut oil), coconut butter is spreadable when soft and becomes hard when chilled. The easiest way I have found to melt hardened coconut butter is to remove the lid, place the jar in a cold oven, and turn the heat to 300 degrees F. As the oven preheats, it will gently soften the coconut butter. After 5 minutes, remove the butter from the oven with a pot holder and stir the contents of the jar. Alternatively, you can stick a jar of coconut butter into an oven that is in the process of cooling down (after you've used the oven for baking). Occasionally, it may be necessary to add a little coconut oil to the jar if its contents seem too dry after melting. Artisana is the most prevalent brand of coconut butter and can be found in health food stores (near either the peanut butters or the oils), some mainstream grocery stores, and online. I've even seen it at Walmart! If you can't find coconut butter or don't want to buy it, there is a tutorial on my website for making your own coconut butter: chocolatecoveredkatie.com/coconut-butter-and-coconut-oil/.

Ground flax: Also known as flaxmeal, ground flax is made from whole flaxseeds ground into a powder. Flaxseeds are high in dietary fiber, protein, and essential omega-3s, -6s, and -9s. But the seeds must be ground for optimal absorption of these nutrients. I often use ground flax in place of eggs to bind ingredients. You can find it in either the bulk aisle or flour section of health food stores and some mainstream grocery stores. Once purchased, ground flax is best stored in an airtight container in the refrigerator or freezer.

Nut butters and allergy-friendly alternatives: For a change of pace, why not try substituting almond butter, cashew butter, or even macadamia nut butter when a recipe calls for peanut butter? Each will contribute its own unique flavor to a dish. If nut allergies are a concern, look into SunButter or NoNuts Golden Peabutter, which are made from sunflower seeds and peas, respectively. A large selection of fancy nut butters can be found in stores like Whole Foods, and many mainstream grocery stores are also beginning to stock a larger selection. My favorite peanut butter is Whole Foods 365 crunchy, but any brand of full-fat peanut butter will work in these recipes, so feel free to use your favorite.

Virgin coconut oil: Coconut oil has been shown to help our bodies fight off viruses and bacteria, regulate thyroid and blood sugar, increase metabolism, and even lower cholesterol. Although high in saturated fat, many studies have proven that saturated fats from vegetable sources do not produce the same negative effects in our bodies as the saturated fats from animal products. Look for virgin—or unrefined—coconut oil, as most refined coconut oil has been bleached and may have had chemicals added during the refining process. My favorite brands are Whole Foods 365 and Trader Joe's, as they are the best-tasting and least-expensive that I've found.

terms to know

Throughout this book, you'll see some language that's worth explaining. When a recipe calls for...

Granulated sugar of choice: Use your choice of the following sugars: coconut sugar, Sucanat, evaporated cane juice sugar, or white sugar.

Sweetener of choice: Use any liquid or granulated sweetener, including pure maple syrup, stevia, coconut sugar, evaporated cane juice, date sugar, and so on. Do keep in mind, however, that some sweeteners (such as pure maple syrup and raw agave) are sweeter than others (such as molasses) and that each sweetener will give each recipe a unique taste. If in doubt, it's best to use the specific sweetener noted in a recipe.

Milk of choice: Use whatever milk you like best. I am partial to almond milk, but hemp milk, oat milk, soy milk, Homemade Dairy-Free Milk (page 134), canned or cartoned coconut milk, or any other type of milk will work.

Canned coconut milk: When a recipe calls specifically for canned coconut milk, don't substitute milk of choice or coconut milk that comes in a carton. Canned coconut milk has a much higher fat content and therefore gives your dessert a richer taste and thicker texture.

Virgin coconut oil: If a recipe in this book calls for coconut *or* vegetable oil, feel free to use your preference. However, in a few cases the recipe will list virgin coconut oil as the sole option. Unlike vegetable oil, virgin coconut oil becomes hard when chilled and therefore must be used to achieve the proper texture in some recipes.

tips, tricks, and troubleshooting

Now that you're armed with all of the necessary information, let's talk about how to use it! Here are some tips and tricks to get you started:

1. When you're making one of these recipes—or any recipe—for the first time, be sure to follow it exactly, right down to the last grain of salt. Do not omit or change anything from the recipe unless you are okay with the possibility that it might not turn out perfectly. Changes to avoid include: substituting a

type of flour not specifically mentioned as an option for a particular recipe, substituting applesauce or yogurt for the oil in a recipe, reducing the oil in a recipe, or reducing the sugar or replacing it with Splenda or stevia baking blend.

However, if you wish to experiment and *understand the possible risks of a subpar result,* please feel free to make changes to a recipe. Edible experiments can be exciting, and you may end up with a new culinary masterpiece of your own!

2. Before you begin cooking, make sure to read through all of the ingredients and instructions. It's never fun to find out you were supposed to soak something overnight when you're already up to your elbows in batter.

3. And do be sure to read the ingredient list carefully. Imitation vanilla is not the same as pure vanilla extract, baking powder is not the same as baking soda, and pancake syrup is not the same as pure maple syrup. If you read through the ingredients thoroughly, these kinds of mix-ups will be easily avoided.

4. Always use the pan size indicated in a recipe. Making a recipe in a pan of a different size may change the baking time, possibly resulting in an overcooked or undercooked dessert.

5. When using measuring cups or spoons, make sure the ingredients are loosely packed and level with the rim of the measuring spoon or measuring cup (unless otherwise stated in a recipe).

6. If using melted coconut oil for a recipe, be sure that any ingredients you mix with it, such as milk or yogurt, are at room temperature. This prevents the coconut oil from solidifying upon contact.

7. Calibrate your oven. Many people are surprised to learn that ovens are often not calibrated correctly. This means if you set your oven to 350 degrees F and put an oven thermometer inside the oven, the number on the thermometer might not actually match the one on your oven's temperature gauge. You can probably imagine how detrimental this discrepancy can be. To calibrate an oven, either follow the directions in your oven's manual or do a quick Google search for "how to calibrate an oven," which will yield numerous step-by-step guides.

8. Finally, remember to take climate into account. Believe it or not, the weather can have a big impact on your baking. In humid weather, flour absorbs less liquid, which can affect the final results. Altitude can also cause variances. In areas of higher elevation, you may need to make changes to certain recipes, such as increasing the baking time.

melting chocolate

One technique that deserves its own mini spotlight is melting chocolate. It can be frustrating if done incorrectly, but it's very simple as long as the right procedure is followed. Below, I've highlighted two of the best methods:

WATER BATH OR DOUBLE BOILER METHOD

Fill the bottom of a medium skillet or double boiler pan with water and bring to a simmer. Place a heatproof bowl or the other half of a double boiler pan on top of the first pan, making sure it sits above (not touching) the water. Fill the top pan with your chocolate pieces.

Keeping the water just below simmering, constantly stir the chocolate until almost melted. Then remove it from the heat and continue to stir until the chocolate is completely melted.

MICROWAVE METHOD

Place the chocolate in a microwave-safe bowl and microwave on 50 percent power for 1 minute (or less if you have just a small amount of chocolate to melt). Stir, then microwave another 30 seconds. Stir again. If the chocolate is still not melted, continue to microwave in 10-second intervals, making sure to stir after each interval.

Tips to keep in mind:

- Begin by breaking any large chunks of chocolate into small ($1/2$-inch or so) pieces.
- Melt the chocolate carefully, slowly, and never on high heat, as it burns quite easily.
- Make sure not to let any water touch the chocolate, as this would cause it to seize.
- Use melted chocolate immediately, as it will re-harden quite quickly.

Now that you know *how* to transform your kitchen into a chocolate-covered paradise, it's time for the fun part: actually making—and, more importantly, *eating*—the desserts!

If you make one of the recipes and want to share your photos or baking experiences, please feel free to post your creations to the Chocolate-Covered Katie Facebook page (facebook.com/chocolatecoveredkatie). I'm always incredibly honored when someone makes one of my recipes, and I'd love to see your results!

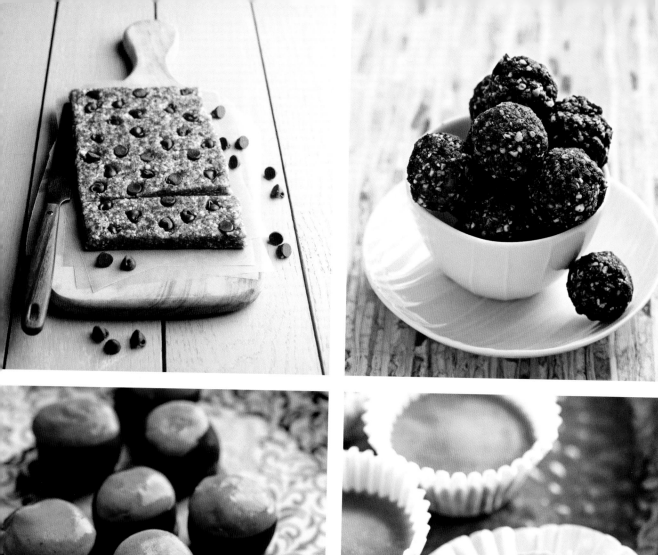

2

cookies, brownies & bars

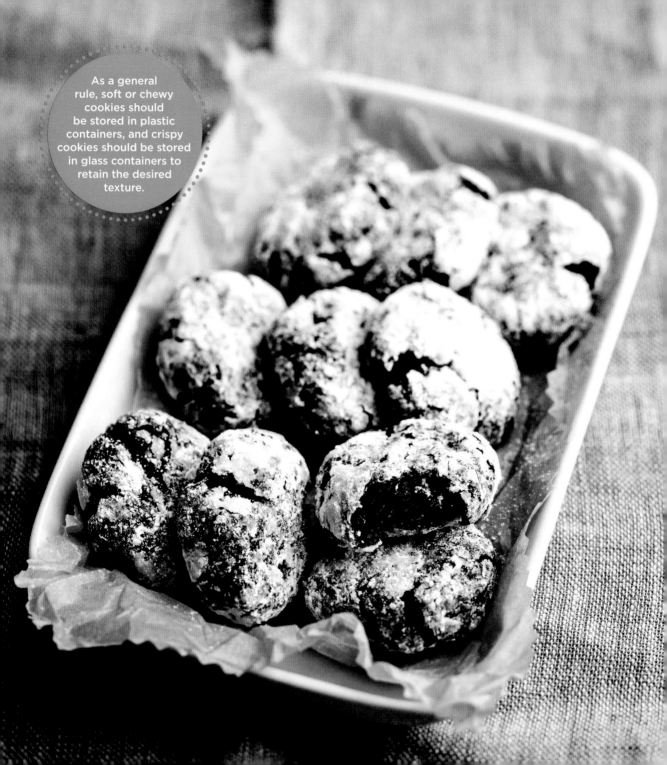

As a general rule, soft or chewy cookies should be stored in plastic containers, and crispy cookies should be stored in glass containers to retain the desired texture.

chocolate pixie cookies

Every Christmas, my grandmother bakes at least ten different types of cookies. And every Christmas, her soft Chocolate Pixies are the overwhelming crowd favorite. I decided to "healthify" the cookies a few years ago, cutting way back on all the fat and sugar. They were so wildly successful that not a single person could tell the difference between the healthier cookies and the originals! makes 20 to 24 cookies

1 cup spelt flour or all-purpose flour*

1/4 cup plus 2 tablespoons cacao powder or unsweetened cocoa powder

1/4 cup plus 2 tablespoons xylitol or granulated sugar of choice

1/4 teaspoon baking soda

1/4 teaspoon salt

1/4 cup vegetable oil or melted coconut oil

3 tablespoons milk of choice

2 tablespoons pure maple syrup or raw agave

1 teaspoon pure vanilla extract

Powdered sugar or Healthier Powdered Sugar (page 188), optional

Lightly grease two baking sheets and set aside.

In a large mixing bowl, combine the flour, cacao powder, sugar of choice, baking soda, and salt and stir very well. In a medium mixing bowl, stir together the oil, milk, maple syrup, and vanilla. Pour wet ingredients into dry and stir to form a dough. Using your hands or a cookie scoop, roll into 20 to 24 balls, then roll in a dish of powdered sugar (if using). Place balls on the prepared baking sheets and refrigerate for 1 hour.

Preheat the oven to 300 degrees F. Bake the chilled balls for 12 minutes. The cookies will look underdone, but they will continue to cook as they cool. Remove from the oven and allow to cool for at least 10 minutes before removing from the sheets. Store leftovers in a covered container at room temperature for up to 3 days.

per cookie

Calories	50	Fat	2.5 grams
Fiber	1.5 grams	Carbs	6.5 grams
Protein	1 gram	Weight Watchers PointsPlus Value	1

*For gluten-free pixie cookies, substitute Bob's Red Mill gluten-free all-purpose baking flour for the flour.

sinless peanut butter cookies

Set a plate of these down at a party and watch them immediately disappear. The recipe was inspired by a childhood favorite called "Sinful Peanut Butter Cookies." But no one should ever make you feel sinful for enjoying dessert…especially when it tastes this good!

makes 24 to 28 cookies

1 cup peanut butter or allergy-friendly alternative

$^{1}/_{4}$ cup applesauce

1 teaspoon pure vanilla extract

$^{3}/_{4}$ cup xylitol or granulated sugar of choice

$^{1}/_{4}$ cup plus 2 tablespoons flour of choice (excluding coconut flour)

1$^{1}/_{2}$ teaspoons baking soda

pinch salt

$^{1}/_{2}$ cup mini chocolate chips, optional

Lightly grease two baking sheets and set aside.

In a medium mixing bowl, whisk together the peanut butter, applesauce, and vanilla until a smooth paste forms. In a small bowl, stir together all remaining ingredients. Pour the dry ingredients into the peanut butter mixture and stir until evenly mixed. Depending on the peanut butter you use, the dough may be too sticky to form balls. If this is the case, freeze the dough for 15 to 20 minutes, until firm.

Using your hands or a cookie scoop, roll or form the dough into 24 to 28 balls and place on the prepared cookie sheets. For soft cookies, refrigerate the dough for 45 minutes or longer before baking. For crispy cookies, proceed directly to the next step.

Preheat the oven to 350 degrees F. Bake the cookies for 8 minutes. The cookies will look underdone, but they will continue to cook as they cool. Remove from the oven and allow to cool for at least 10 minutes before removing from the sheet. Store leftovers in a covered container at room temperature for up to 3 days.

per cookie

Calories	65	Fat	4 grams
Fiber	1 gram	Carbs	4.5 grams
Protein	2.5 grams	Weight Watchers PointsPlus Value	2

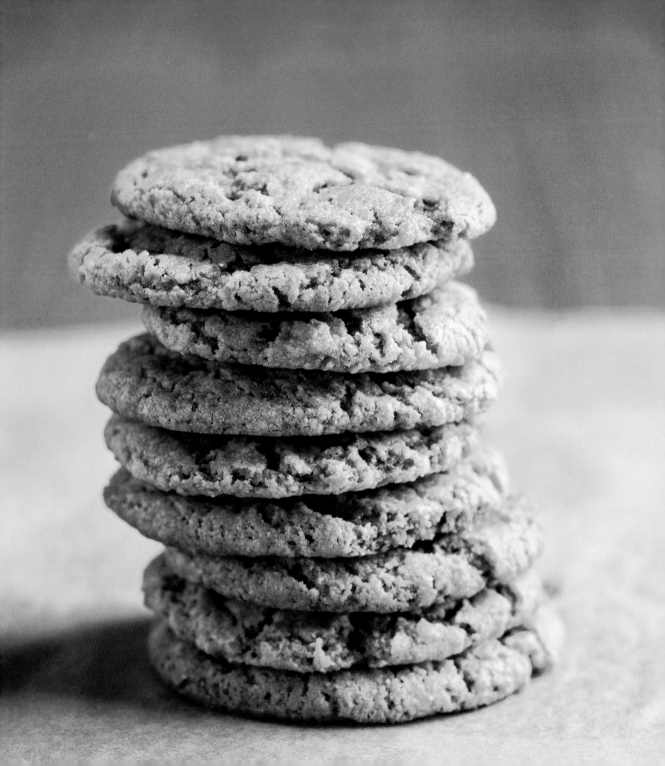

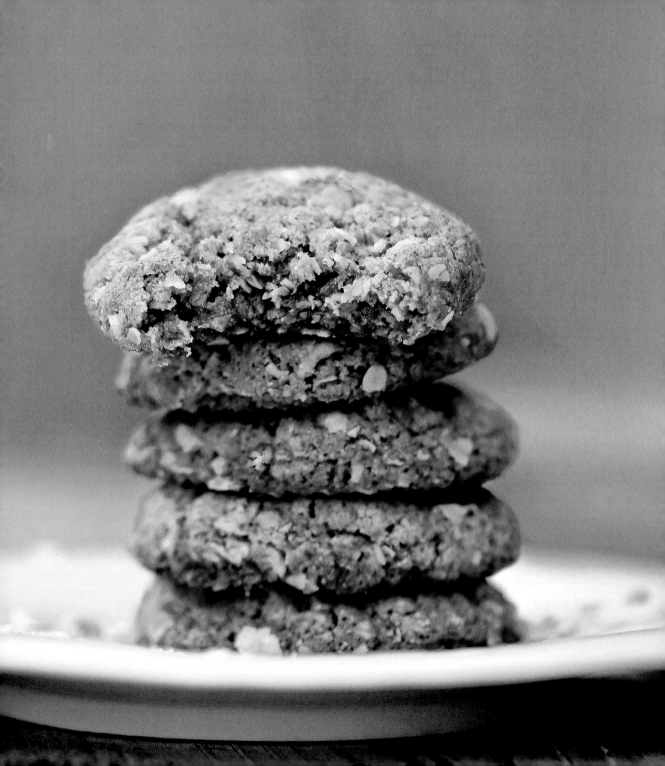

chewy oatmeal crinkle cookies

With rolled oats, whole grains, and omega-3-rich flax, these hearty oatmeal cookies are so healthy you could get away with eating them for breakfast. Haven't you always wanted to eat cookies for breakfast?

makes 15 to 20 cookies

- 3½ tablespoons vegetable oil or melted coconut oil
- 2 tablespoons milk of choice
- 1 tablespoon ground flax
- ¼ teaspoon pure vanilla extract
- ¾ cup quick-cooking oats
- ½ cup spelt flour or all-purpose flour*
- ½ cup brown sugar, date sugar, or coconut sugar
- ⅜ teaspoon baking soda
- ¼ teaspoon salt
- pinch pure stevia extract, or 1 tablespoon granulated sugar of choice

Line a baking sheet with parchment paper and set aside. In a small mixing bowl, whisk together the oil, milk, ground flax, and vanilla. Allow to sit for at least 5 minutes. In a large mixing bowl, combine all remaining ingredients and stir very well. Pour wet ingredients into dry and stir until a dough forms. Transfer dough to a gallon-sized resealable plastic bag and smush into a big ball. Remove dough from the bag. Using your hands or a cookie scoop, roll or form the dough into 15 to 20 balls and place on the prepared baking sheet about 2 inches apart. Freeze for 15 minutes, or refrigerate for 4 hours. The dough balls can also be frozen for up to a month. When ready to bake, preheat the oven to 350 degrees F. For chewy cookies, bake for 8 minutes. For crispy cookies, bake for 10 minutes. The cookies will look underdone at first, but this is what you want; they continue to cook as they cool. Remove from the oven and allow to cool for at least 10 minutes before removing from the sheet. Store leftovers in a covered container at room temperature for up to 3 days.

per cookie

Calories	55		Fat	2.5 grams
Fiber	1 gram		Carbs	7.5 grams
Protein	1 gram	Weight Watchers PointsPlus Value	1

*For gluten-free oatmeal cookies, substitute Bob's Red Mill gluten-free all-purpose baking flour for the flour.

flourless chocolate chip cookies

Sophomore year of college, I lived in a tiny apartment with a closet-sized kitchen. Luckily I had the best roommate in the world, and we loved nothing more than to come home from class, drop our books at the door, and head straight to our ~~closet~~ kitchen to bake cookies. The chocolate chip cookies below are a product of one such baking session, and we liked them so much that both of us still make the recipe, seven years later! **makes 24 to 28 cookies**

---

3 cups rolled oats

$1/2$ cup brown sugar, date sugar, or coconut sugar

1 teaspoon baking soda

$1/2$ teaspoon salt

$1/2$ cup chocolate chips

$1/4$ cup plus 2 tablespoons xylitol or granulated sugar of choice

$1/4$ cup vegetable oil or melted coconut oil

4 to 6 tablespoons milk of choice

Preheat the oven to 375 degrees F. Lightly grease two baking sheets and set aside.

Blend together the oats, brown sugar, baking soda, and salt in a blender or food processor until evenly combined. Place in a large mixing bowl and add chocolate chips, sugar of choice, oil, and 2 tablespoons of the milk. Stir together to form a dough, very slowly adding more milk of choice if the mixture is too dry to form a dough. Using your hands or a cookie scoop, roll or form into 24 to 28 balls. Place on the prepared sheets, then press the balls to flatten.

Bake for 6 minutes. The cookies will look underdone at first, but this is what you want; the cookies continue to cook as they cool. Remove from the oven and allow to cool for at least 10 minutes before removing from the sheets. Store leftovers in a covered container at room temperature for up to 3 days.

per cookie

Calories	75	Fat	3 grams
Fiber	1 gram	Carbs	10 grams
Protein	1.5 grams	Weight Watchers PointsPlus Value	2

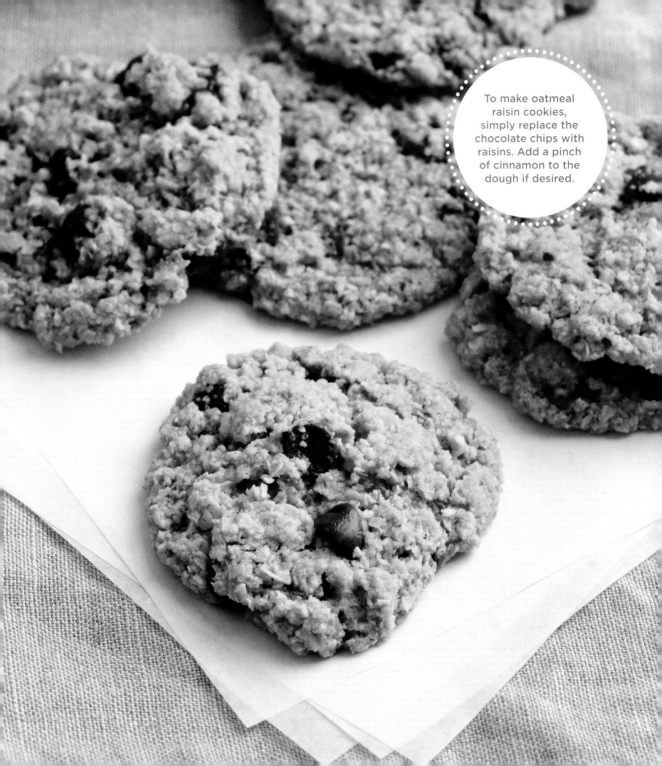

To make oatmeal raisin cookies, simply replace the chocolate chips with raisins. Add a pinch of cinnamon to the dough if desired.

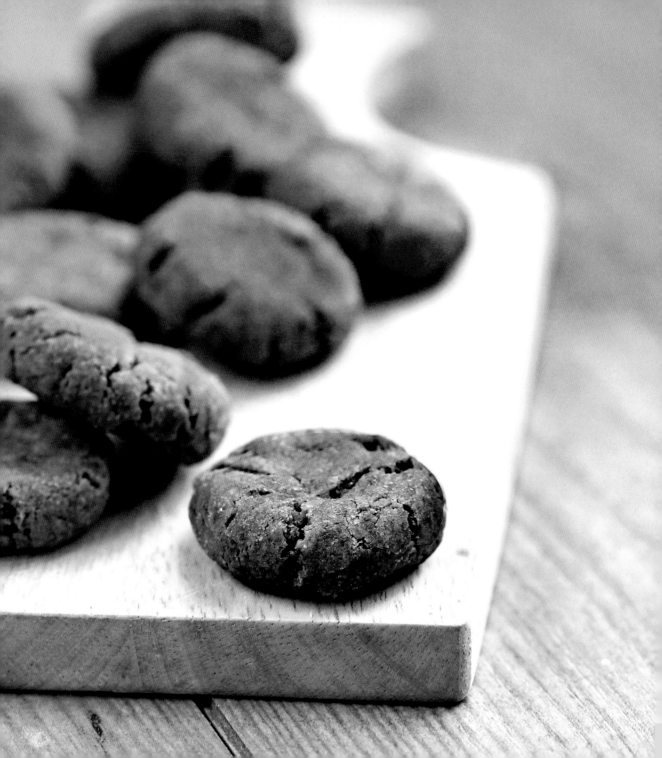

gingerbread molasses cookies

Delightfully chewy and incredibly soft, this is the perfect cookie recipe to share with your best friends. makes 15 to 18 cookies

---

$^2/_3$ cup oat flour (see page 17)

$^1/_3$ cup spelt flour or all-purpose flour*

$^1/_3$ cup Sucanat or brown sugar

$^1/_2$ teaspoon baking soda

$^1/_2$ teaspoon baking powder

$^1/_2$ teaspoon ginger

$^1/_4$ teaspoon cinnamon

$^1/_4$ teaspoon salt

$2^1/_2$ tablespoons vegetable oil or melted coconut oil

2 tablespoons applesauce

1 tablespoon molasses

$^1/_2$ teaspoon pure vanilla extract

Line a large plate with parchment paper and set aside.

In a large mixing bowl, combine the flours, Sucanat, baking soda, baking powder, ginger, cinnamon, and salt and stir very well. In a medium mixing bowl, whisk together all remaining ingredients. Pour wet ingredients into dry and mix with a spoon until mostly incorporated.

Transfer the crumbly dough to a gallon-sized resealable plastic bag and smush it into one big ball. Open the bag and, using your hands or a cookie scoop, break off small pieces and roll into 15 to 18 balls. Place balls on the prepared plate. Refrigerate for at least 1 hour. Dough balls can also be frozen for up to a month.

When ready to bake, preheat the oven to 350 degrees F. Slide the parchment paper—with the cookies—onto a baking sheet and bake for 10 minutes. Remove from the oven and press the cookies down. The cookies will look underdone at first, but this is what you want; the cookies continue to cook as they cool. Allow to cool for at least 10 minutes before removing from the sheet. Store at room temperature for up to 3 days. For soft cookies, store in a plastic container; for crispier cookies, store in a glass container.

per cookie

Calories	50	Fat	2 grams
Fiber	1 gram	Carbs	7.5 grams
Protein	1 gram	Weight Watchers PointsPlus Value	1

*For gluten-free gingerbread cookies, substitute Bob's Red Mill gluten-free all-purpose baking flour for the flour.

chocolate-covered thin mintz

These taste just like the Girl Scout cookies you know and love, but without any of those unhealthy artificial ingredients or trans fats. The recipe is dedicated to anyone who has ever eaten an entire box of Thin Mints in a single sitting. I can't be the only one, right?

makes about 24 cookies

COOKIES
1/4 cup plus 2 tablespoons spelt flour or all-purpose flour

3 tablespoons Dutch-processed cocoa powder

3 tablespoons xylitol or granulated sugar of choice

1/8 teaspoon baking soda

1/8 teaspoon salt

2 tablespoons vegetable oil

1 1/2 tablespoons milk of choice

1 tablespoon pure maple syrup

1/2 teaspoon pure vanilla extract

1/8 teaspoon pure peppermint extract

CHOCOLATE COATING
3 1/2 tablespoons cacao powder or unsweetened cocoa powder

2 1/2 tablespoons virgin coconut oil, melted (see box on opposite page)

1 tablespoon pure maple syrup

1/4 teaspoon pure peppermint extract

For the cookies: In a large mixing bowl, combine the flour, cocoa powder, sugar of choice, baking soda, and salt and stir very well. In a medium mixing bowl, whisk together all remaining cookie ingredients. Pour wet ingredients into dry and stir to form a dough. Refrigerate dough at least 1 hour.

Preheat the oven to 300 degrees F. Lightly grease two baking sheets and set aside.

Transfer the chilled dough to a gallon-sized resealable plastic bag and smush hard to form a ball. While the dough is still in the bag, roll it out with a rolling pin until it fills the bag.

Entirely cut away one side of the bag so that the dough is exposed. Using a round cookie cutter or a lid, cut out rounds from the dough and transfer to the prepared baking sheets.

Bake the cookies for 10 minutes. They will look underdone at first, but this is what you want; they continue to cook as they cool. Remove from the oven and allow to cool for at least 10 minutes before removing from the sheets.

For the chocolate coating: Line a large plate with parchment or waxed paper and set aside. Combine all ingredients in a long, shallow dish.

Stir until the texture resembles that of chocolate sauce.

Dunk the edges of each cooled cookie into the chocolate, then spread chocolate over the top of each cookie with a spoon. Place the cookies on the prepared plate and refrigerate for at least 20 minutes so that the coating sets. These cookies are best stored in a covered container in the refrigerator, as the coconut coating will soften when warm. They will last up to a week refrigerated.

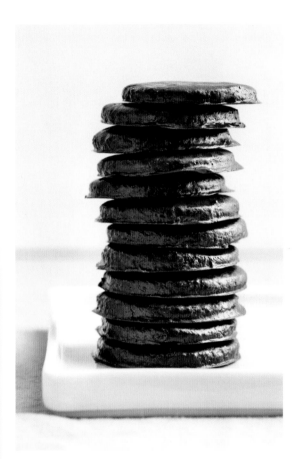

Recipe Substitutions

This recipe has many possible substitutions: Regular unsweetened cocoa powder may be substituted for the Dutch-processed cocoa powder. The cookies will still be delicious, but they will taste a little less authentic. Additionally, coconut oil can be substituted for the vegetable oil in the dough. You will need to roll out the dough and cut the circles *before* chilling the dough if you opt for the coconut-oil version. Finally, for a coconut-free coating, simply melt ½ cup chocolate chips with ½ teaspoon pure peppermint extract and 1 teaspoon non-hydrogenated shortening (such as Spectrum brand).

per cookie, with coating

Calories	35	Fat	2.5 grams
Fiber	1 gram	Carbs	3.5 grams
Protein	.5 gram	Weight Watchers PointsPlus Value	1

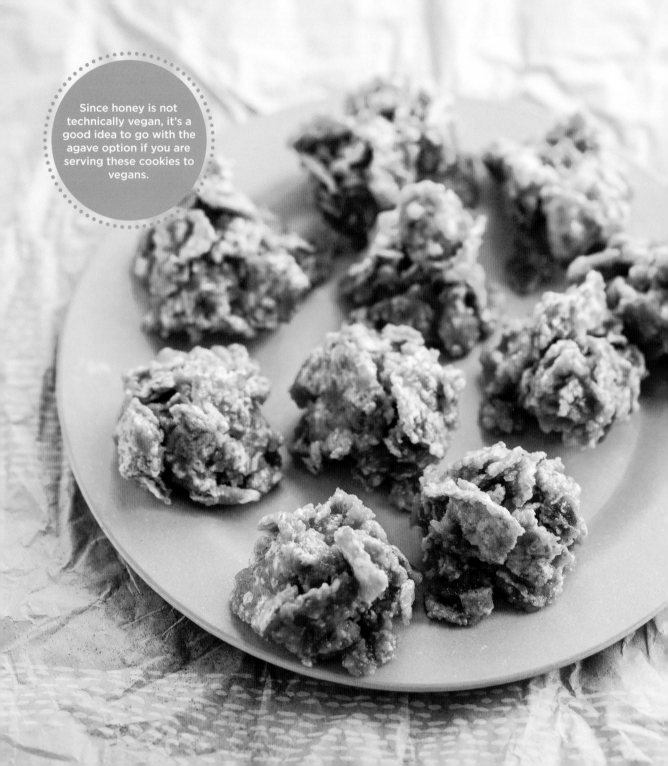

Since honey is not technically vegan, it's a good idea to go with the agave option if you are serving these cookies to vegans.

special cck no-bake cookies

Dating back to the 1950s, the popular Special K no-bake cookie recipe traditionally included an entire cup of both white sugar *and* corn syrup. Here is my healthier answer to those Special K treats. They offer fiber, iron, and potassium while still being just as addictive as the originals.

makes about 27 cookies

---

1 cup peanut butter or allergy-friendly alternative

¼ cup raw agave or honey (see note on opposite page)

2 tablespoons applesauce

1 tablespoon molasses

3 tablespoons xylitol or granulated sugar of choice

⅛ teaspoon salt

4 cups bran flakes (I like Whole Foods 365 brand), or gluten-free alternative

---

Line two large plates with parchment or waxed paper and set aside.

In a large mixing bowl, stir together the peanut butter, agave, applesauce, and molasses until completely smooth. Add the sugar of choice and salt and stir to incorporate.

Pour the bran flakes into the mixture and stir very well until the flakes are evenly coated. It's okay if some flakes break during the process. Using two spoons or your hands, form into clusters and set on the prepared plates.

Cover and freeze for 8 hours, until firm. Store leftovers in a sealed container for up to a week in the freezer.

per cookie

Calories	80	Fat	4.5 grams
Fiber	2.5 grams	Carbs	10 grams
Protein	3 grams	Weight Watchers PointsPlus Value	2

secretly healthy brownies

Each bite is so decadently fudgy you'd never guess these bold brownies are cholesterol-free, gluten-free, dairy-free, low in sugar, *and* high in omega-3s and fiber. One of my friends proclaimed this to be the best brownie recipe he's ever tried, healthy or not! makes 20 to 24 brownies

BROWNIES
1 cup water

2/3 cup vegetable oil or melted coconut oil

1/2 cup applesauce

2 tablespoons ground flax

2 teaspoons pure vanilla extract

1 cup coconut flour (see page 16)

3/4 cup cacao powder or unsweetened cocoa powder

3/4 cup xylitol or granulated sugar of choice

1/2 teaspoon baking soda

1/2 teaspoon salt

1/16 teaspoon pure stevia extract, or additional 2 tablespoons granulated sugar of choice

CHOCOLATE FROSTING
1/2 cup melted virgin coconut oil

1/2 cup cacao powder or unsweetened cocoa powder

2 tablespoons pure maple syrup or raw agave

For the brownies: Preheat the oven to 350 degrees F. Line a 9x13-inch baking pan with parchment paper and set aside.

In a medium mixing bowl, whisk together the water, oil, applesauce, flax, and vanilla. In a large mixing bowl, combine all remaining brownie ingredients and stir very well. Pour the wet ingredients into the dry and stir until evenly mixed. Transfer the batter to the prepared baking pan. Using a full sheet of parchment or waxed paper, press down very firmly until the brownie batter evenly covers the pan. Remove before cooking.

Bake for 24 minutes, until mostly firm. Remove from the oven and pat down hard with a pancake spatula or another sheet of parchment paper. Refrigerate the pan overnight, as the brownies will not only firm up considerably during this time, they will also taste much sweeter and more chocolaty.

For the frosting: Stir all the ingredients together until a sauce forms.

Frost the brownies with the frosting. Refrigerate the brownies for 10 minutes to set the frosting.

Remove the brownies from the refrigerator and cut into squares. As a general rule, cutting brownies with a plastic knife, and wiping it between each cut, prevents crumbling. These brownies are best stored in the refrigerator or

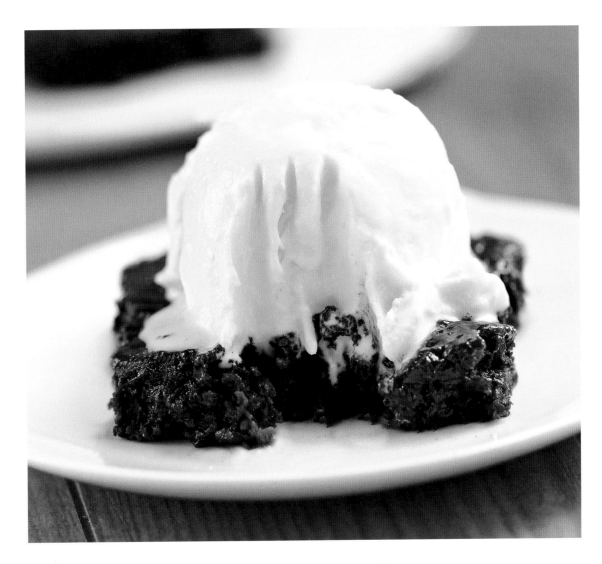

freezer. Refrigerate leftovers in a covered container for up to 4 days, or freeze for up to a month. The brownie in the photo is topped with Pure Bliss Vanilla Ice Cream (page 106).

per frosted brownie

Calories	85	Fat	6.5 grams
Fiber	3 grams	Carbs	6 grams
Protein	2 grams	Weight Watchers PointsPlus Value	2

double chocolate peppermint brownies

This tried-and-true brownie recipe stands up to any boxed brownie mix. The concept of beans in a brownie may sound strange at first, but you will be pleasantly surprised! They're bound to convert your entire family. **makes 9 to 12 brownies**

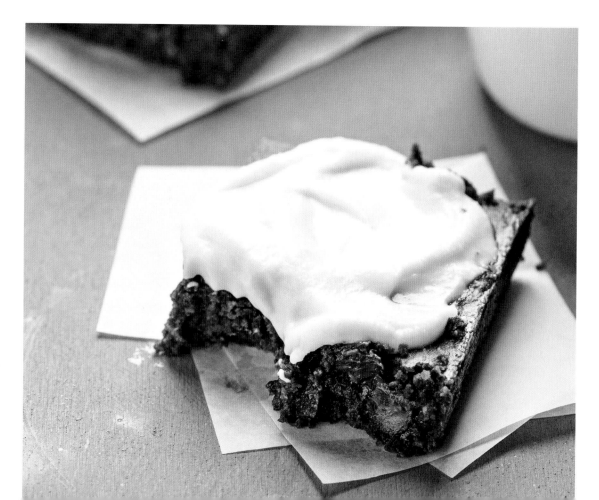

BROWNIES

1 (15-ounce) can black beans, drained and rinsed well

½ cup quick-cooking oats

⅓ cup pure maple syrup

¼ cup vegetable oil or melted coconut oil

3 tablespoons cacao powder or unsweetened cocoa powder

2½ teaspoons pure vanilla extract

½ teaspoon baking powder

¼ teaspoon salt

1/16 teaspoon pure stevia extract, or 2 tablespoons granulated sugar of choice

½ to ⅔ cup chocolate chips, plus more for topping the brownies if desired

YOGURT FROSTING

½ cup plain yogurt (I like WholeSoy or So Delicious cultured coconut milk)

¼ cup melted coconut butter

2 tablespoons powdered sugar or Healthier Powdered Sugar (page 188)

¼ teaspoon pure peppermint extract

For the brownies: Preheat the oven to 350 degrees F. Grease an 8-inch square pan and set aside.

In a high-quality food processor (a blender is not recommended here, but see Note), process all brownie ingredients, except chocolate chips, until completely smooth. Turn off the food processor and stir in the chocolate chips.

Transfer the batter to the prepared pan. If desired, sprinkle additional chocolate chips on top. Bake the brownies for 16 minutes, until firm. Remove from the oven and allow to cool at least 30 minutes before cutting into squares. If brownies are still too fudgy for your liking, cover and refrigerate overnight. They will firm up during this time.

For the frosting: Let the yogurt come to room temperature, or gently warm it for a few seconds in a microwave. This will prevent the melted coconut butter from clumping. Just before serving, mix all the frosting ingredients together in a small bowl and spread over the cut brownies. Refrigerate for 10 minutes, until the frosting hardens.

Refrigerate leftovers in a covered container for up to 4 days. If possible, make these brownies the day before serving, as they taste twice as sweet and chocolaty the next day!

Note: **If you must use a blender for this recipe, blend the batter in two batches, which gives all the ingredients a chance to evenly blend. This is the only way to achieve the correct texture.**

per frosted brownie

Calories	120	Fat	5.5 grams
Fiber	3 grams	Carbs	15 grams
Protein	2.5 grams	Weight Watchers PointsPlus Value	3

the ultimate unbaked brownies

A quick recipe for those days when you just *really* need a brownie. And if you're anything like me, that would be every day. Good thing these babies freeze well! **makes 16 to 20 brownies**

2½ cups loosely packed pitted dates

1½ cups walnuts

6 tablespoons plus ¼ cup cacao powder or unsweetened cocoa powder, divided

1½ teaspoons plus ½ teaspoon vanilla extract, divided

2 teaspoons water

⅜ teaspoon salt

¼ cup pure maple syrup

2 tablespoons vegetable oil or melted coconut oil

Combine the dates, nuts, the 6 tablespoons cacao powder, 1½ teaspoons of the vanilla, the water, and the salt in a high-quality food processor. Process until completely smooth.

Lightly grease an 8-inch square baking dish, or line with parchment or waxed paper. Transfer the dough to the baking dish and press very firmly into the pan with your hands until the dough evenly covers the pan.

In a medium mixing bowl, combine the remaining ¼ cup cacao powder, the remaining ½ teaspoon vanilla, the maple syrup, and the oil and stir to form a paste. Spread the paste evenly over the dough in the pan.

Refrigerate for at least 2 hours to set, then cut into squares. Refrigerate leftovers in a covered container for up to 2 weeks, or freeze for up to 2 months.

per frosted brownie

Calories	140		Fat	7 grams
Fiber	3.5 grams		Carbs	20 grams
Protein	3.5 grams		Weight Watchers PointsPlus Value	4

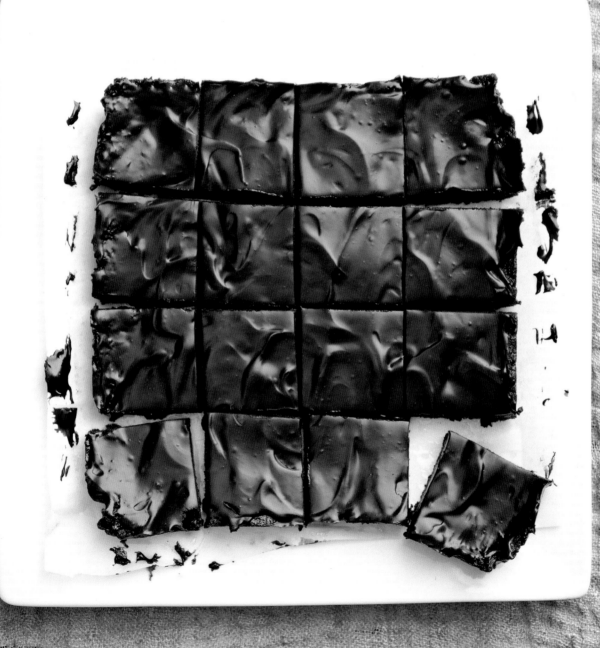

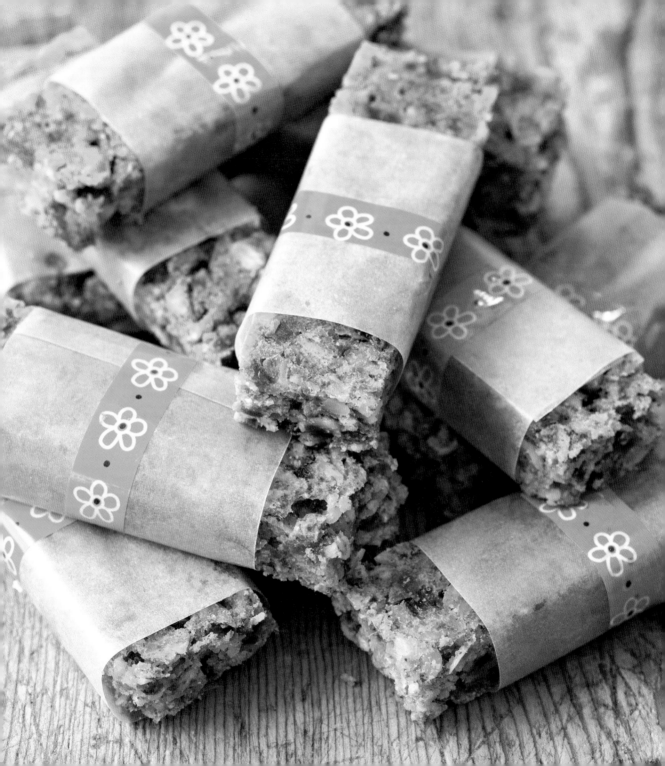

pumpkin pie granola bars

Sweetened with real fruit, these wholesome granola bars are one snack you can feel *good* about giving to your children. That is…if you're willing to share. Try them either unfrosted or iced with melted coconut butter. makes 20 to 22 bars

1 cup canned pumpkin or pumpkin puree

½ cup almond butter (roasted, with salt) or allergy-friendly alternative

1½ teaspoons pure vanilla extract

¼ cup packed dried apricots (about 7 apricots)

½ cup dried cranberries or dried cherries

½ cup raw almonds

1 cup puffed wheat or puffed rice

1 cup rolled oats

½ teaspoon pumpkin pie spice

½ teaspoon cinnamon

$3/8$ teaspoon salt

$1/16$ heaping teaspoon pure stevia extract, or 3 tablespoons granulated sugar of choice

Preheat the oven to 350 degrees F. Line a 10-inch square baking pan with parchment or waxed paper and set aside.

In a medium bowl, stir together the pumpkin and almond butter until smooth. Stir in the vanilla and set aside. In a high-quality food processor, process the dried fruit and almonds until they form fine crumbles. Transfer to a large mixing bowl and stir in the puffed wheat, oats, pumpkin pie spice, cinnamon, salt, and sweetener.

Add the almond butter mixture to the large bowl and stir until evenly combined. Pour batter into the prepared baking pan, smoothing evenly. Cover with another sheet of parchment paper and press down very firmly. Remove before baking.

Bake for 30 to 35 minutes, until firm. Remove from the oven and allow to cool for at least 15 minutes in the pan. Press down very firmly again before slicing into bars. Refrigerate leftovers in a covered container for up to a week, or freeze for up to a month.

per granola bar

Calories	75	Fat	3.5 grams
Fiber	2 grams	Carbs	8 grams
Protein	2.5 grams	Weight Watchers PointsPlus Value	2

chocolate raspberry crumble bars

With gooey melted chocolate, sweet red raspberries, and a buttery crumble crust, these bars always go fast when you bring them to a party, and they're great for barbecues and picnics as well. People constantly beg me for the recipe, so I knew I had to include it in this book. You can switch out the raspberries for chopped strawberries or cherries if you'd like. makes 12 to 16 bars

$1\frac{1}{2}$ cups spelt flour or all-purpose flour*

$\frac{1}{2}$ teaspoon baking powder

$\frac{3}{4}$ teaspoon salt

$\frac{1}{4}$ cup xylitol or granulated sugar of choice

$\frac{1}{16}$ teaspoon pure stevia extract, or additional 2 tablespoons granulated sugar of choice

$\frac{1}{4}$ cup vegetable oil or melted coconut oil

3 tablespoons milk of choice

2 cups raspberries (fresh or thawed frozen)

$\frac{1}{2}$ cup chocolate chips

3 tablespoons pure maple syrup

2 teaspoons pure vanilla extract

1 tablespoon cornstarch or arrowroot

Preheat the oven to 350 degrees F. Lightly grease an 8x8-inch baking dish or line with parchment paper and set aside.

In a large mixing bowl, combine the flour, baking powder, salt, and dry sweeteners and stir very well. Add the oil and milk and stir until a dough forms. Transfer half the dough to the baking dish and press down very firmly with a spatula.

In another large mixing bowl, combine the raspberries, chocolate chips, maple syrup, vanilla, and cornstarch. Stir well. Pour this mixture evenly over the dough in the baking dish.

Sprinkle the remaining dough over the baking dish and press down lightly. Bake for 45 minutes, until firm. Remove from the oven and allow to cool for at least 15 minutes in the pan before slicing into bars. Refrigerate leftovers in a covered container for up to 4 days.

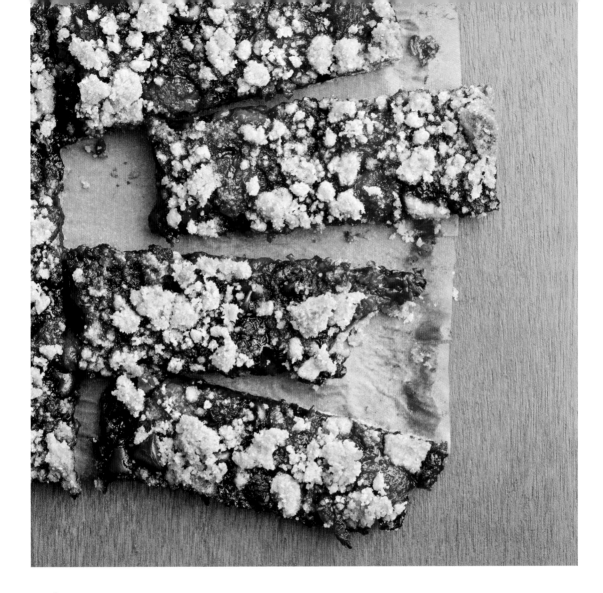

per bar

Calories	100	Fat	5 grams
Fiber	3 grams	Carbs	13 grams
Protein	2.5 grams	Weight Watchers PointsPlus Value	3

*For gluten-free bars, substitute Bob's Red Mill gluten-free all-purpose baking flour for the flour and add ½ teaspoon xanthan gum with the flour.

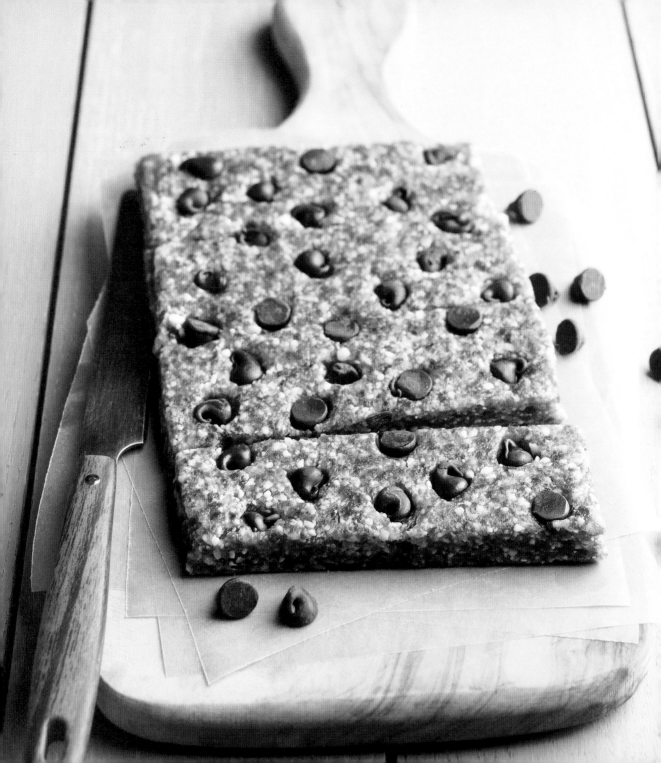

i ♥ chocolate chip cookie dough bars

I am slightly obsessed with cookie dough. (Understatement!) Ever since the day I learned that you can omit the egg from a chocolate chip cookie recipe and eat the raw dough to your heart's content, life has never been the same. So a recipe for actual bars of homemade cookie dough pretty much has my name written all over it. **makes 12 bars**

3 cups packed pitted dates

1½ cups raw nuts of choice

1½ teaspoons pure vanilla extract

½ teaspoon salt

1 ounce chocolate bar of choice, optional

chocolate chips or homemade chocolate chips (see page 198) for garnish

In a high-quality food processor, blend all the ingredients except the chocolate chips until a fine crumble forms. If the mixture is too dry, add up to 1 tablespoon water. Divide the dough evenly between 2 gallon-sized resealable plastic bags and smush each into a ball. With the dough still inside a bag, use a rolling pin to roll it out until it fills up the entire bag. Repeat with the second bag.

Cut away the top sides of the bags so that the dough is exposed. Using a knife or a cookie cutter, cut into bars. Press a few chocolate chips into each bar if desired. Store leftovers in a covered container at room temperature for up to 3 days, refrigerate for up to 2 weeks, or freeze for up to 2 months.

per bar

Calories	220	Fat	9 grams
Fiber	5.5 grams	Carbs	40 grams
Protein	4 grams	Weight Watchers PointsPlus Value	7

carrot cake bars with coconut frosting

There are less than 100 calories in each of these carrot cake bars. And that includes the frosting! makes 18 to 20 bars

CARROT CAKE BARS
1 cup spelt flour or all-purpose flour*

$\frac{1}{4}$ cup xylitol or granulated sugar of choice

$\frac{1}{8}$ teaspoon pure stevia extract, or additional $\frac{1}{4}$ cup granulated sugar of choice

2$\frac{1}{2}$ teaspoons cinnamon

1 teaspoon baking powder

$\frac{1}{2}$ teaspoon baking soda

$\frac{1}{2}$ teaspoon salt

$\frac{1}{2}$ cup finely chopped walnuts, optional

$\frac{1}{2}$ cup raisins, optional

1$\frac{1}{4}$ cups steamed and sliced carrots, or 1 cup carrot puree

$\frac{1}{4}$ cup milk of choice

$\frac{1}{4}$ cup vegetable oil or melted coconut oil (see opposite page)

2 tablespoons ground flax

1 tablespoon pure vanilla extract

COCONUT FROSTING
1 small banana, mashed

$\frac{1}{4}$ cup plus 2 tablespoons melted coconut butter

$\frac{3}{4}$ teaspoon pure vanilla extract

$\frac{1}{16}$ teaspoon salt

shredded coconut, optional

For the bars: Preheat the oven to 350 degrees F. Lightly grease a 9x13-inch baking pan and set aside.

In a large mixing bowl, combine the flour, sweetener(s), cinnamon, baking powder, baking soda, salt, and walnuts and raisins (if using).

Process the carrots, milk, oil, flax, and vanilla in a blender or food processor until smooth. (Alternatively, mash the carrots until smooth and whisk together with the milk, oil, flax, and vanilla.) Pour wet ingredients into dry and stir until just evenly combined. Transfer the batter to the prepared pan.

Bake for 15 minutes, until firm. Remove from the oven and allow to cool at least 15 minutes before frosting.

For the frosting: Stir together the banana, coconut butter, vanilla, and salt until completely smooth. Spread evenly over the cooled carrot cake bars, then sprinkle with shredded coconut, if desired. Cut into bars, using a plastic knife for no crumbling.

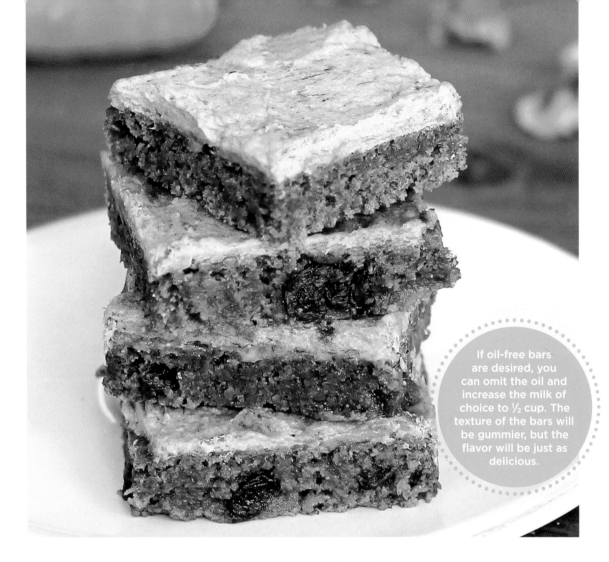

If oil-free bars are desired, you can omit the oil and increase the milk of choice to ½ cup. The texture of the bars will be gummier, but the flavor will be just as delicious.

Place the bars in the refrigerator for at least 2 hours, until the frosting hardens. Refrigerate leftovers in a covered container for up to 3 days.

per frosted bar

Calories	80	Fat	5.5 grams
Fiber	2 grams	Carbs	7 grams
Protein	1.5 grams	Weight Watchers PointsPlus Value	2

*For gluten-free bars, substitute Bob's Red Mill gluten-free all-purpose baking flour for the flour and add ½ teaspoon xanthan gum with the flour.

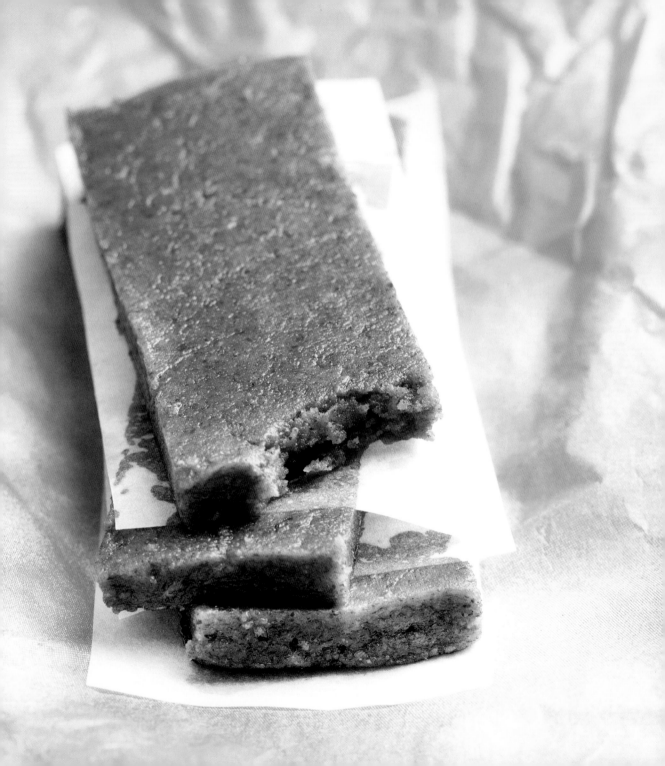

real-food protein bars

Have you looked at the labels of the protein bars on the market these days? Most have such a long list of processed ingredients you might start to wonder if they're even food at all. Do your body a favor and make your own protein bars instead, with less than 10 ingredients.

makes 12 to 16 bars

1 cup almond butter (roasted, with salt) or allergy-friendly alternative

1/4 cup mashed banana or applesauce

1/2 cup vanilla protein powder of choice (I like rice protein powder from Nutribiotic)

1/4 cup Sucanat or brown sugar

1 1/2 teaspoons baking soda

1 teaspoon cinnamon

1/8 teaspoon salt

In a medium mixing bowl, stir together the almond butter and banana until a smooth paste forms, making sure no lumps are present. In a separate medium mixing bowl, stir together all remaining ingredients. Combine the contents of the two bowls and stir until evenly incorporated, resulting in a crumbly dough.

Divide the dough evenly between 2 gallon-sized resealable plastic bags and smush each to form a ball. With the dough still inside the bags, use a rolling pin to roll it out to about a 1/4-inch thickness. Cut away the top sides of the bags so that the dough is exposed. Using a knife, cut into bars. Transfer the bars to a plate or container, cover, and freeze for at least 5 hours, until firm. Once firm, the bars may be stored in a covered container in the refrigerator for up to 1 week, or in the freezer for up to 1 month.

per protein bar

Calories	135	Fat	8 grams
Fiber	2 grams	Carbs	9 grams
Protein	8 grams	Weight Watchers PointsPlus Value	4

chocolate peanut butter buckeyes

Recipes for these melt-in-your-mouth confections, named for their resemblance to the nut of the Ohio buckeye tree, are traditionally overloaded with butter and sugar. In this healthier version, I cut out the butter and significantly reduce the sugar without sacrificing any of the flavor. **makes about 20 buckeyes**

$3/4$ cup peanut butter or allergy-friendly alternative*

$1/2$ cup powdered sugar or Healthier Powdered Sugar (page 188)

$1/4$ heaping teaspoon salt

2 tablespoons cacao powder or unsweetened cocoa powder

2 tablespoons melted virgin coconut oil

$1 1/2$ teaspoons pure maple syrup

Line a large plate with parchment or waxed paper and set aside.

In a medium mixing bowl, stir together the peanut butter, powdered sugar, and salt until a crumbly dough forms (see note below). Transfer the dough to a gallon-sized resealable plastic bag and smush into a big ball. Open the bag and roll the dough into about 20 balls. Place on the prepared plate and freeze for 1 hour, until firm.

In a shallow dish, mix together the cacao powder and melted coconut oil. Stir in the maple syrup, and continue stirring until it looks like chocolate sauce. Remove one ball from the freezer, keeping the rest cold. Using a corn-cob skewer or fork, submerge the ball in the chocolate sauce to coat. Immediately return the covered ball to the freezer. Repeat with the remaining balls, returning them to the freezer to harden for at least 10 minutes.

Store frozen until ready to serve. Leftovers will keep in the freezer for up to a month.

per buckeye

Calories	75		Fat	6 grams
Fiber	1 gram		Carbs	3 grams
Protein	2.5 grams	Weight Watchers PointsPlus Value	2	

*Different brands of peanut butter will yield different textures, so add more peanut butter if the dough is too dry, or add more powdered sugar if it's too gooey.

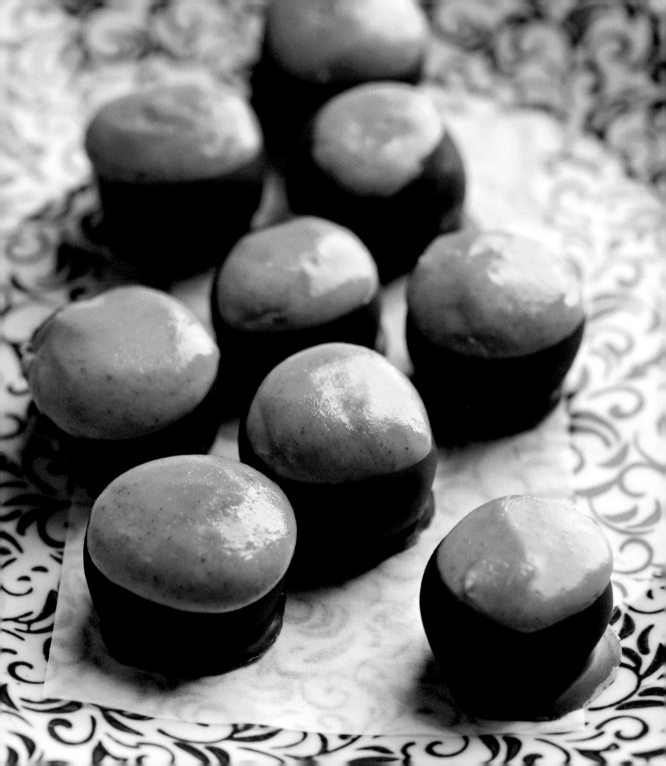

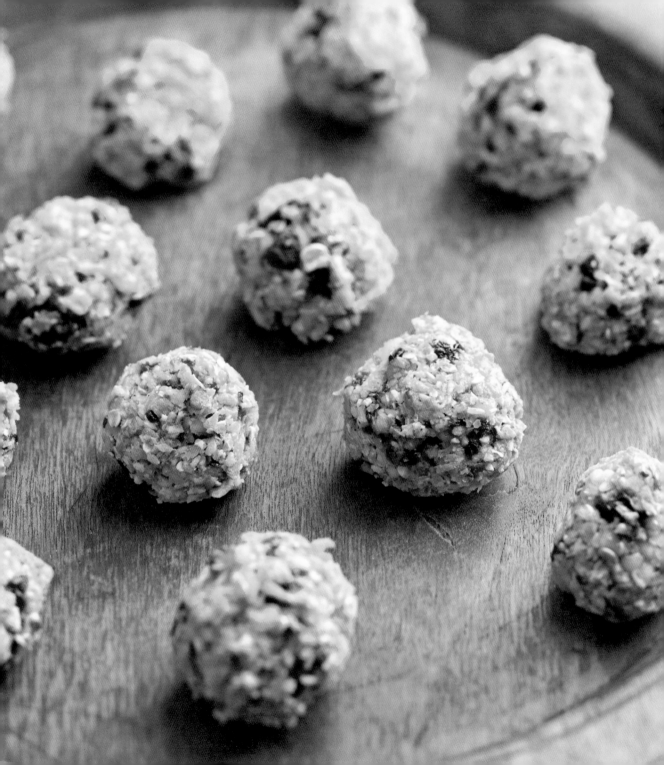

carrot raisin cookie bites

Take your carrot cake on the go with these cookies. They are almost as adorable as they are delicious. Kids will love rolling the dough into balls, and everyone loves popping these bite-sized cookies straight into their mouths! **makes 14 to 16 bites**

1 small carrot, peeled and cut into coins

$\frac{1}{2}$ cup raisins

$\frac{1}{2}$ cup walnuts

$\frac{1}{4}$ cup plus 2 tablespoons quick-cooking oats

$\frac{1}{4}$ teaspoon cinnamon

$\frac{1}{8}$ teaspoon plus $\frac{1}{16}$ teaspoon salt

$\frac{1}{4}$ cup shredded coconut, optional

Combine all ingredients in a high-quality food processor and process very well.

Transfer the mixture to a gallon-sized resealable plastic bag and smush into a ball. Open the bag and shape the dough into about 15 balls, using your hands or a cookie scoop.

Refrigerate in a covered container for up to 2 weeks, or freeze for up to 2 months.

per bite

Calories	45		Fat	2.5 grams
Fiber	1 gram		Carbs	5.5 grams
Protein	1.5 grams	Weight Watchers PointsPlus Value	1	

anytime chocolate fudge balls

It's impossible to eat just one! These simple fudge balls need no refrigeration and are great for lunch boxes, road trips, and on-the-go snacking. Walnuts may be substituted for the pecans, and the coconut can easily be omitted if you prefer. makes 10 to 14 balls

³/₄ cup pitted dates

½ cup raw pecans

2 tablespoons cacao powder or unsweetened cocoa powder

2 tablespoons shredded coconut

½ teaspoon pure vanilla extract

¹/₁₆ teaspoon salt

1 handful mini chocolate chips, optional

Combine all ingredients in a high-quality food processor and process until a fine crumble forms. If the mixture is too dry, add up to 1 tablespoon water.

Transfer the dough to a gallon-sized resealable plastic bag and smush into a ball. Open the bag, break off pieces of dough, and roll into balls.

Store in a covered container at room temperature for up to 3 days, refrigerate for up to 2 weeks, or freeze for up to 2 months.

per fudge ball

Calories	45	Fat	2 grams
Fiber	2 grams	Carbs	8 grams
Protein	.5 gram	Weight Watchers PointsPlus Value	1

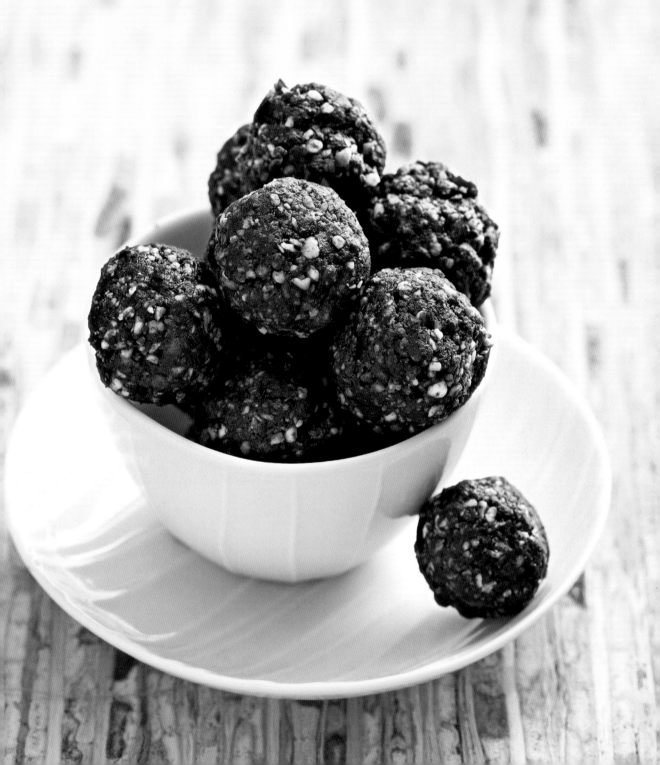

peanut butter & jelly candy cups

Having lived in Japan for much of my childhood, I was well-versed in sushi, soba, and yakitori. But I never tried a single peanut butter and jelly sandwich until the fifth grade! When a friend finally did introduce me to the salty-sweet combination, I was mesmerized and could not get enough. In the following recipe, I've given the celebrated childhood sandwich a candy-inspired makeover. Just be glad I didn't include miso soup... **makes 8 to 10 peanut butter cups**

level ½ cup powdered peanut butter (see box on opposite page)

¼ cup virgin coconut oil or cacao butter, melted

4 teaspoons pure maple syrup

3 tablespoons jam of choice (I like St. Dalfour strawberry)

Line the cups of a mini muffin tin with mini cupcake liners and set aside.

In a small bowl, combine the powdered peanut butter, coconut oil, and maple syrup. Stir to form a paste.

Place just under 1 teaspoon of the mixture into each mini cupcake liner. Freeze for 10 minutes, until firm to the touch.

Divide the jam evenly among the liners and top with the remaining peanut butter mixture. Freeze for 15 minutes, until solid.

If you used coconut oil, keep these peanut butter cups refrigerated or frozen. If you used cacao butter, the candies can be stored at room temperature. Store in a covered container for up to a month.

per candy cup

Calories	75	Fat	6 grams
Fiber	2 grams	Carbs	5 grams
Protein	2 grams	Weight Watchers PointsPlus Value	2

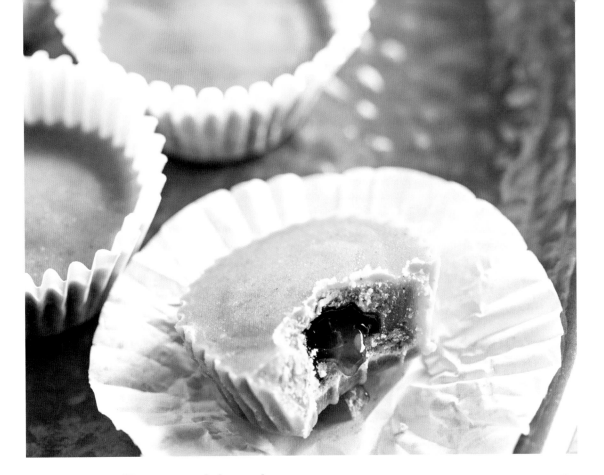

Peanut Butter Version

If you can't find powdered peanut butter or would prefer to use the real thing in this recipe, try this variation:

¼ cup peanut butter

1 tablespoon virgin coconut oil, melted

pinch salt

½ teaspoon pure vanilla extract

1½ teaspoons pure maple syrup

3 tablespoons jam of choice

Follow the same directions as in the main recipe.

Powdered Peanut Butter

Powdered peanut butter is made by squeezing the oils out of peanuts and dehydrating the remaining product, yielding a lower calorie count. Powdered peanut butter is sold in many grocery stores as well as online. The most popular brands include PB2 from Bell Plantation and Just Great Stuff brand from Betty Lou's.

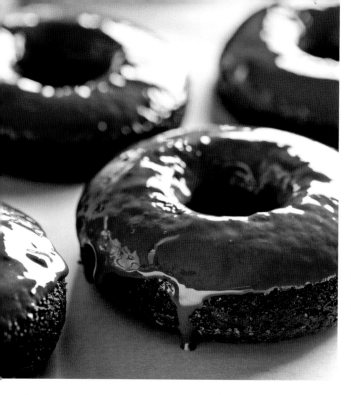

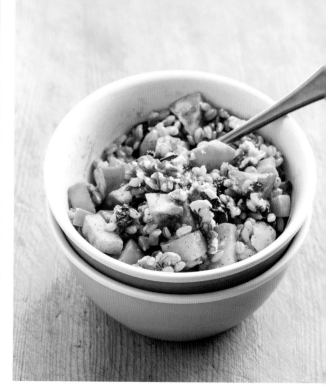

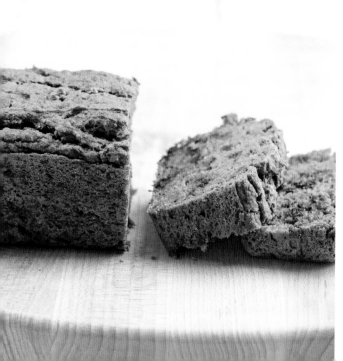

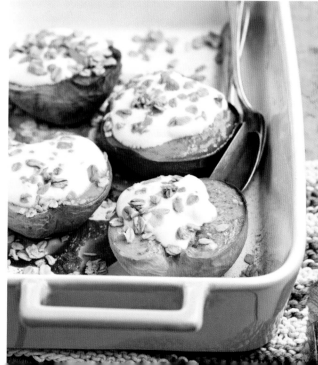

3

dessert
for
breakfast

chocolate brownie waffles

Do you consider yourself a chocoholic? Do you think about chocolate all day, go to bed craving chocolate, dream about eating chocolate, and wake up craving chocolate? If so, these waffles are for you!

makes 4 waffles

1 cup spelt flour or all-purpose flour

1/4 cup plus 2 tablespoons cacao powder or unsweetened cocoa powder

1 1/2 teaspoons baking powder

1/4 teaspoon baking soda

1/4 teaspoon salt

1/8 teaspoon pure stevia extract, or 1/4 cup sweetener of choice

scant 1 cup milk, or 3/4 cup if using a liquid sweetener as your choice above

1 tablespoon plus 2 teaspoons vegetable oil or melted coconut oil

1 tablespoon plus 1 teaspoon pure vanilla extract

Grease a waffle iron and preheat it as needed.

In a small bowl, combine the flour, cacao powder, baking powder, baking soda, salt, and stevia (or other sweetener, if using) and mix well. In a separate bowl, combine the liquid sweetener (if using), milk, oil, and vanilla.

Pour the wet ingredients into the dry and stir to combine. Using about one-fourth of the batter, follow instructions specific to your machine to make a waffle. Repeat to make 4 waffles, greasing the waffle iron after each waffle.

Serve with pure maple syrup, or top with fresh berries and Coconut Whipped Cream (page 183). Or go all out: brownie waffles à la mode!

per waffle

Calories	170	Fat	8 grams
Fiber	7 grams	Carbs	26 grams
Protein	6 grams	Weight Watchers PointsPlus Value	5

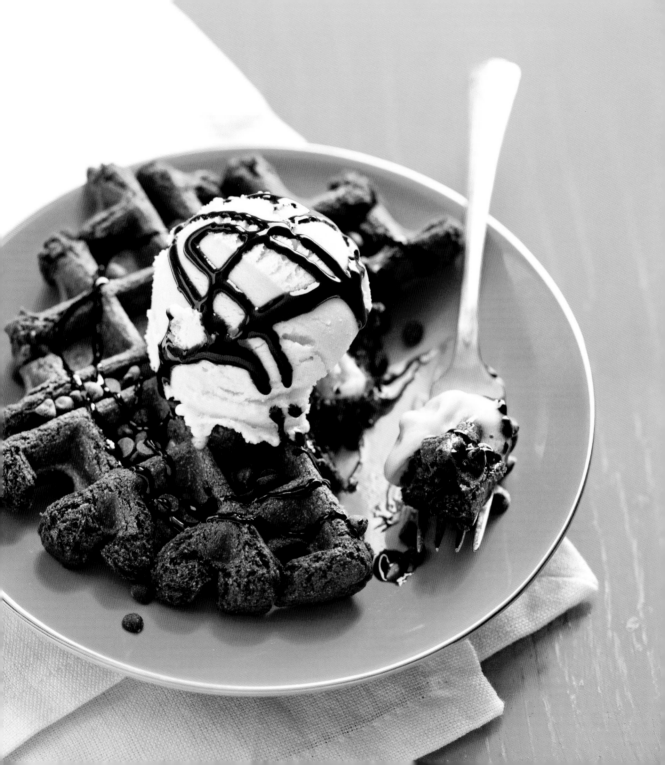

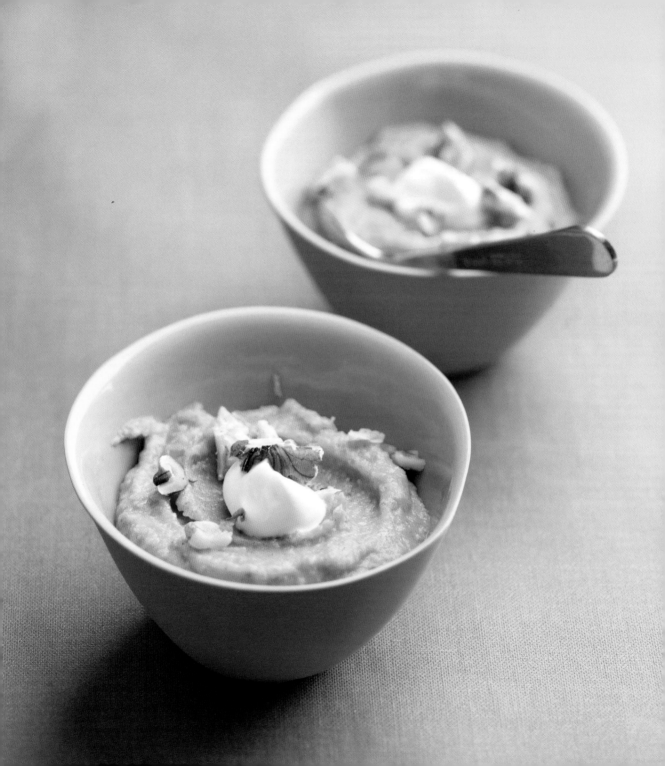

pumpkin breakfast pudding

If your mornings are rushed and you often find yourself without the time to cook an elaborate meal, here is a satisfying breakfast recipe that might just be the perfect solution. It's quick, easy to make, and it literally tastes like you are eating a big bowl of pumpkin pie without the crust. makes 2 servings

---

²/₃ cup canned pumpkin or pumpkin puree

2 cups flake cereal, such as bran flakes or corn flakes

1¹/₂ cups milk of choice

1 teaspoon pure vanilla extract

¹/₂ teaspoon cinnamon

¹/₄ teaspoon salt

sweetener of choice, to taste

handful chopped walnuts or pecans, optional

handful dried fruit of choice, optional

In a blender or Magic Bullet, blend the pumpkin, cereal, milk, vanilla, cinnamon, salt, and sweetener until completely smooth.

Taste, then add additional sweetener if desired. Stir in nuts and dried fruit if using. Refrigerate 20 to 30 minutes, until the mixture thickens to the consistency of pudding.

Heat or serve cold. Top with Coconut Whipped Cream (page 183), if desired.

per serving

Calories	175	Fat	3 grams
Fiber	8 grams	Carbs	28 grams
Protein	7 grams	Weight Watchers PointsPlus Value	4

blueberry morning baked oatmeal

On those cold winter mornings when your family craves something hearty and comforting, this berry-stuffed oatmeal is a welcome addition to the breakfast table. It will keep everyone happily full for hours.

makes 4 to 6 servings

2½ cups blueberries (fresh or thawed frozen)

1 cup rolled oats

⅔ cup plus ½ cup milk of choice

3 to 6 tablespoons sweetener of choice, depending on desired sweetness

1/16 teaspoon pure stevia extract, or additional 2 tablespoons sweetener of choice

3½ tablespoons vegetable oil or melted coconut oil (see note on opposite page)

3 tablespoons ground flax

2 teaspoons pure vanilla extract

½ teaspoon salt

½ cup shredded coconut, optional

½ teaspoon cinnamon, optional

Preheat the oven to 375 degrees F. Lightly grease an 8-inch square baking pan and set aside.

Combine the blueberries and rolled oats in a bowl. Pour evenly into the prepared pan.

In a mixing bowl, whisk together ⅔ cup milk and all remaining ingredients (reserving the remaining ½ cup milk). Spread this mixture evenly over the blueberry layer and stir quickly. Top with the reserved milk.

Bake for 35 minutes, until golden. Remove from the oven and allow to sit for 5 minutes before cutting into slices using a knife or a large cookie cutter. Serve topped with fresh blueberries and pure maple syrup, if desired. Refrigerate leftovers in a covered container for up to 3 days, or freeze for up to a month.

per serving

Calories	160		Fat	6 grams
Fiber	5 grams		Carbs	18 grams
Protein	3 grams	Weight Watchers PointsPlus Value		3

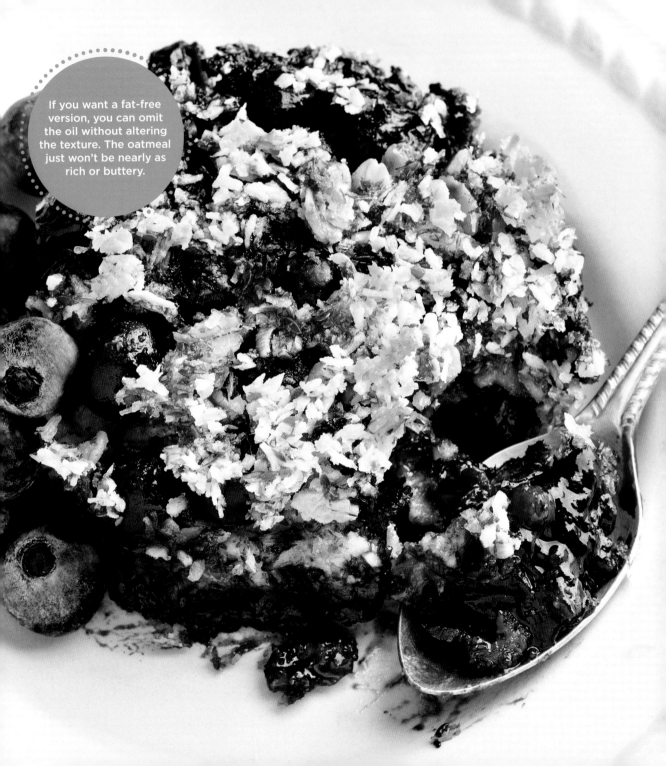

If you want a fat-free version, you can omit the oil without altering the texture. The oatmeal just won't be nearly as rich or buttery.

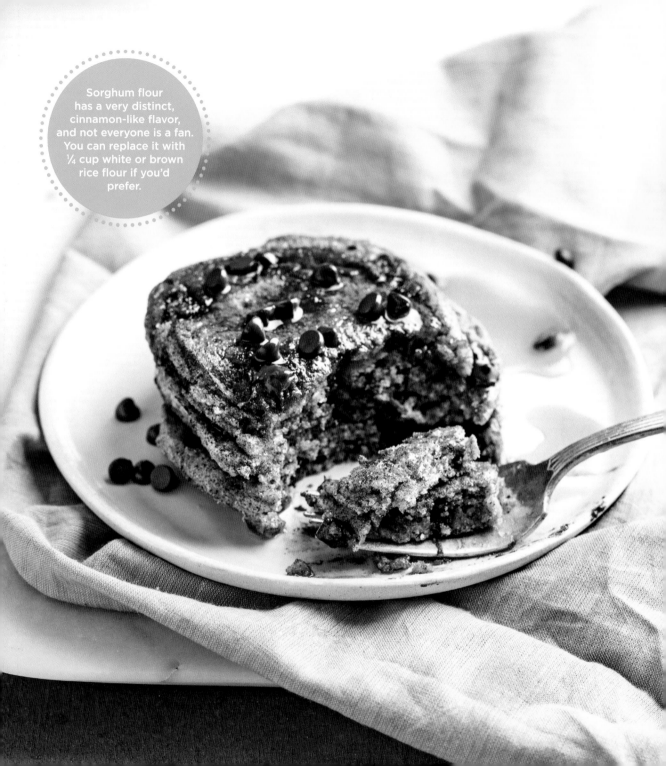

Sorghum flour has a very distinct, cinnamon-like flavor, and not everyone is a fan. You can replace it with ¼ cup white or brown rice flour if you'd prefer.

gluten-free chocolate chip pancakes

This recipe is dedicated to my childhood best friend. One morning after a sleepover, she requested chocolate chip pancakes when her father asked what we wanted to eat. The notion that chocolate could be eaten for breakfast completely rocked my world...and I've never looked back. makes 10 to 11 pancakes

---

1/4 cup sorghum flour (see note on opposite page)

2 tablespoons buckwheat flour

2 tablespoons potato starch

2 to 4 tablespoons chocolate chips or mini chocolate chips

1 teaspoon baking powder

1/4 teaspoon baking soda

3/8 teaspoon salt

1/16 teaspoon pure stevia extract, or 2 tablespoons pure maple syrup

1/2 cup applesauce

1/3 cup milk of choice, or 1/4 cup if using maple syrup instead of stevia

1 teaspoon pure vanilla extract

In a medium mixing bowl, combine the flours, potato starch, chocolate chips, baking powder, baking soda, salt, and stevia (if using). Stir together very well. In a separate medium mixing bowl, whisk together the 1/4 cup maple syrup (if using), applesauce, milk, and vanilla. Pour dry ingredients into wet, and stir together to form a batter.

Lightly grease a medium skillet and place over medium heat. Test the heat of your skillet by throwing a few drops of water onto the surface; when the water sizzles, the pan is ready for the pancake batter. Drop small ladlefuls (about 3 tablespoons each) of batter onto the skillet and cook until the edges begin to look dry. Immediately flip the pancakes, using a spatula, and cook an additional minute, until golden brown. If the pancakes brown too quickly, lower the heat slightly. Repeat with remaining batter, greasing the skillet each time.

Top with pure maple syrup or anything else your heart desires!

per pancake

Calories	35	Fat	1 gram
Fiber	1 gram	Carbs	7 grams
Protein	1 gram	Weight Watchers PointsPlus Value	1

elvis peanut butter pancakes

Take my hand, take my whole heart too... You won't be able to help falling in love with these wholesome peanut butter pancakes.

makes 14 silver-dollar pancakes

1/2 cup mashed banana

2 tablespoons peanut butter or allergy-friendly alternative

1 teaspoon pure vanilla extract

1/2 cup plus 2 tablespoons

water, or 1/2 cup if using a liquid sweetener instead of stevia

2 tablespoons liquid sweetener of choice, or 1/16 teaspoon pure stevia extract

1/3 cup spelt flour or all-purpose flour

1 1/2 teaspoons baking powder

1/2 teaspoon salt

In a small bowl, combine the banana, peanut butter, vanilla, water, and 2 tablespoons liquid sweetener (if using instead of stevia) and stir until a paste forms. In a separate small bowl, combine the flour, baking powder, salt, and stevia (if using) and stir well.

Pour dry ingredients into wet, and stir together to form a batter.

Lightly grease a medium skillet and place over medium heat. Test the heat of your skillet by throwing a few drops of water onto the surface; when the water sizzles, the pan is ready for the pancake batter. Drop small ladlefuls (about 3 tablespoons each) of batter onto the skillet. Cook until the edges begin to look dry. Immediately flip pancakes, using a spatula, and cook an additional minute, until golden brown. If the pancakes brown too quickly, lower the heat slightly. Repeat with remaining batter, greasing the skillet each time. Serve with your favorite toppings, such as pure maple syrup or peanut butter and sliced bananas.

per pancake

Calories	25	Fat	1 gram
Fiber	1 gram	Carbs	3.5 grams
Protein	1 gram	Weight Watchers PointsPlus Value	1

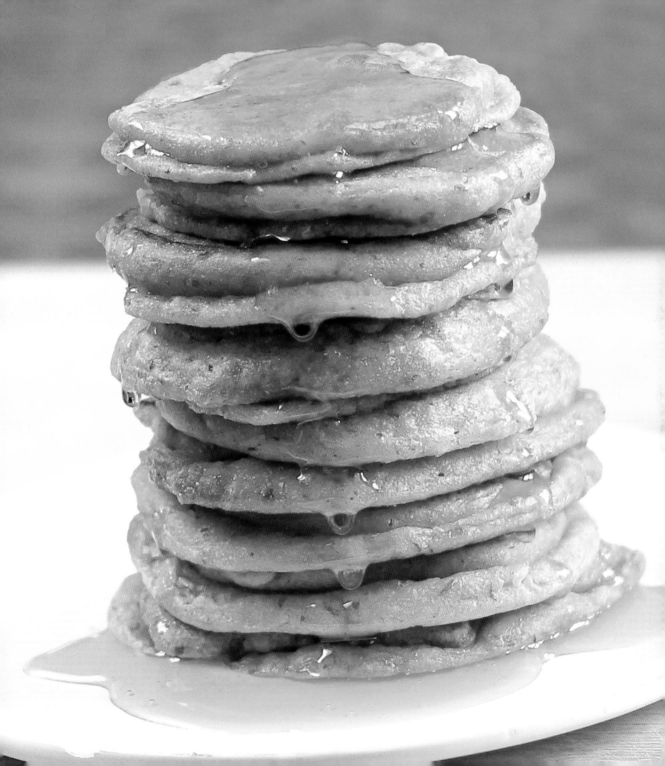

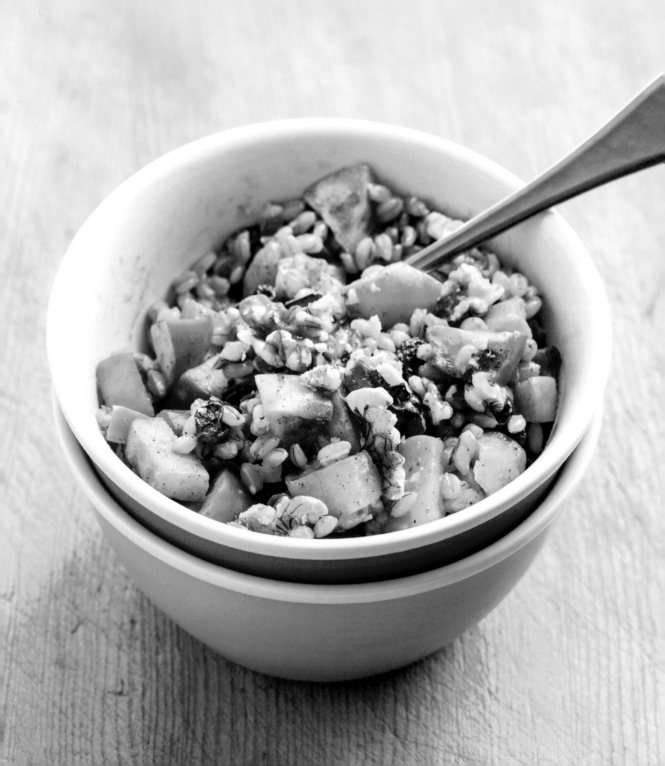

the "no more hunger" breakfast bowl

Cold cereal just does not fill me up. Whenever I eat it for breakfast, I'm hungry again 3 seconds later. This nutritious hot cereal, on the other hand, has some serious staying power, keeping me full for hours. It's high in fiber, magnesium, and protein, and each spoonful is like eating a giant oatmeal cookie, straight from the oven. **makes 2 to 3 servings**

½ cup hulled barley

2¼ cups water

½ teaspoon salt, plus more if needed

2 chopped apples, peeled if desired

½ cup raisins

1 teaspoon cinnamon

¼ cup milk of choice

1 teaspoon pure vanilla extract

sweetener of choice, to taste

crushed walnuts, optional

In a medium saucepan, cover the barley with water and let soak overnight. Drain, then pour barley back into the saucepan. Add 2 cups of the water and the salt and bring to a boil over high heat. Cover, reduce the heat to low, and simmer for at least 2 hours, until thick and fluffy. Drain through a fine mesh strainer to remove excess liquid.

In a separate small saucepan, combine the remaining ¼ cup water, the apples, raisins, and cinnamon. Cook over medium heat until the water is mostly absorbed and the apple is soft. Add the softened barley, milk, and vanilla. Sweeten to taste. Add a pinch of salt and top with crushed walnuts, if desired.

per serving

Calories	250	Fat	1 gram
Fiber	10 grams	Carbs	55 grams
Protein	5 grams	Weight Watchers PointsPlus Value	5

superfood
chocolate bowls

With more potassium and almost twice the amount of fiber as other grains, quinoa is a complete protein, containing *all nine* essential amino acids. This decadent chocolate hot cereal is so filling that you won't even blink when those sugary breakfast pastries come your way. And you can feel good knowing you nourished your body with a healthy and satisfying meal. makes 4 servings

- 1 cup uncooked quinoa, rinsed
- 3 cups milk of choice
- $^3/_8$ teaspoon salt
- $^1/_4$ cup cacao powder or unsweetened cocoa powder
- 1 tablespoon pure vanilla extract
- sweetener of choice, to taste
- mini chocolate chips, optional
- 1 large banana, mashed, optional
- 3 tablespoons peanut butter, optional
- coconut milk for serving, optional

In a medium saucepan, bring the quinoa, milk, and salt to a boil. Cover, turn the heat to low, and cook for 30 minutes, until the quinoa is soft and fluffy.

Turn off the heat and stir in the cacao powder, vanilla, and desired sweetener. Mix in the chocolate chips, mashed banana, and/or peanut butter if using. Top with coconut milk, if desired.

per serving

Calories	180		Fat	5 grams
Fiber	6 grams		Carbs	30 grams
Protein	7.5 grams		Weight Watchers PointsPlus Value	5

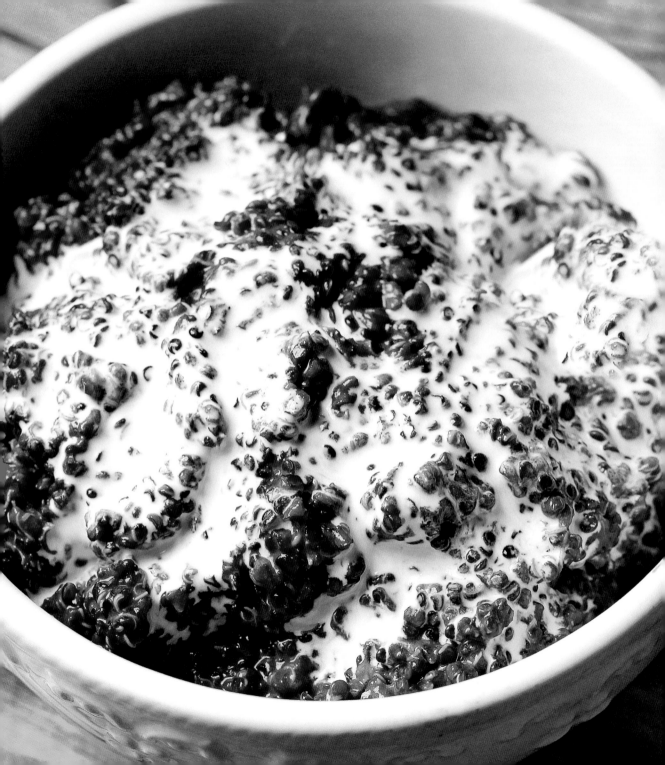

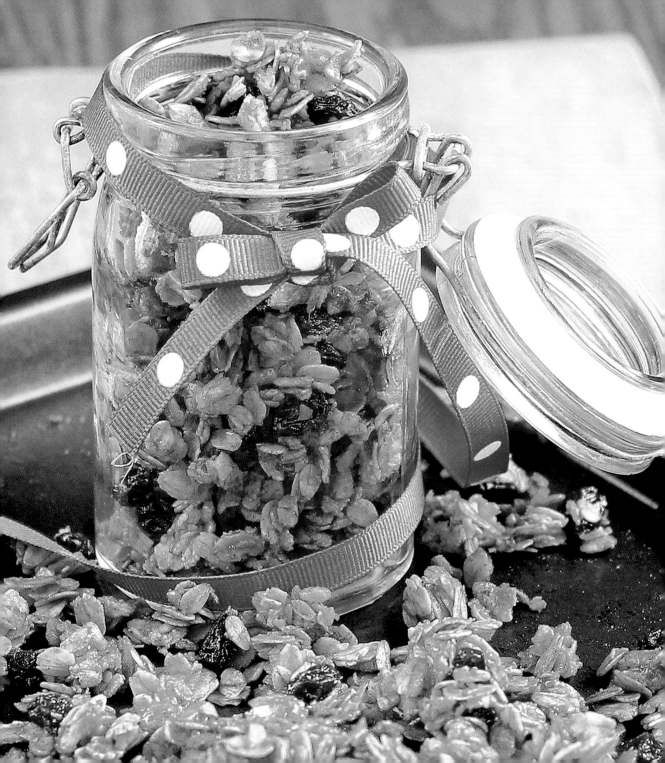

cinnamon raisin granola

Sprinkle this sweet cinnamon granola over yogurt, cereal, or even ice cream. Once you make your own granola, it's almost impossible to imagine going back to store-bought. **makes about 2½ cups (5 servings)**

1 cup rolled oats

¼ cup brown or white crisped rice cereal, gluten-free if desired

3 tablespoons pure maple syrup or raw agave

2 tablespoons vegetable oil or melted coconut oil

½ teaspoon pure vanilla extract

½ teaspoon cinnamon

¼ teaspoon baking soda

¼ teaspoon salt

pinch pure stevia extract, or 1 tablespoon sweetener of choice

¼ to ½ cup raisins

Preheat the oven to 350 degrees F. Line a baking sheet with parchment paper and set aside.

In a large mixing bowl, combine all ingredients except the raisins and stir until combined. Spread out the granola mixture in a thin layer on the prepared baking sheet and bake for 5 minutes. Using a spoon or spatula, flip the granola. Bake for an additional 2 minutes. Remove from the oven and set aside for 10 minutes, allowing the granola to become crispy as it cools.

Add the raisins and stir until evenly mixed. Leftovers can be stored at room temperature in a covered container for up to 3 weeks.

Make This Recipe Your Own!

- Substitute dried cranberries or dried cherries for the raisins.

- Add ½ cup slivered almonds before baking.

- Add ½ cup shredded coconut after baking.

- Substitute rolled spelt flakes, Kamut flakes, or barley flakes for the oats.

Experiment and have fun with it!

per ½-cup serving

Calories	70	Fat	5 grams
Fiber	2 grams	Carbs	25 grams
Protein	2.5 grams	Weight Watchers PointsPlus Value	4

midnight chocolate crunch granola

Whether it's seven o'clock in the morning or twelve at night, there is absolutely no wrong time to eat chocolate. Try this devilishly healthy granola layered in a breakfast parfait, or enjoy by the handful as a late-night snack. **makes about 2½ cups (5 servings)**

1 cup rolled oats

⅓ cup chopped or slivered almonds

2 tablespoons cacao powder or unsweetened cocoa powder

⅛ teaspoon salt

pinch pure stevia extract, or 1 tablespoon granulated sugar of choice

3 tablespoons vegetable oil or melted coconut oil

2 tablespoons pure maple syrup or raw agave

1 teaspoon pure vanilla extract

⅓ cup freeze-dried raspberries

¼ cup raisins

⅓ cup chocolate chips or homemade chips (see page 198), optional

Preheat the oven to 350 degrees F. Line a baking sheet with parchment paper and set aside.

In a large mixing bowl, combine the oats, almonds, cacao powder, salt, and sweetener of choice and stir. Add the oil, maple syrup, and vanilla, and stir until combined. Spread out mixture in a thin layer on the prepared baking sheet and bake for 15 minutes. Flip the granola, using a spoon or spatula, and bake for an additional 5 minutes. Remove from the oven and set aside for 10 minutes, allowing the granola to become crispy as it cools.

Stir in the raspberries and raisins. When the granola has cooled completely, stir in the chocolate chips, if desired. Leftovers can be stored at room temperature in a covered container for up to 3 weeks.

per ½-cup serving

Calories	200	Fat	12 grams
Fiber	6 grams	Carbs	25 grams
Protein	5 grams	Weight Watchers PointsPlus Value	6

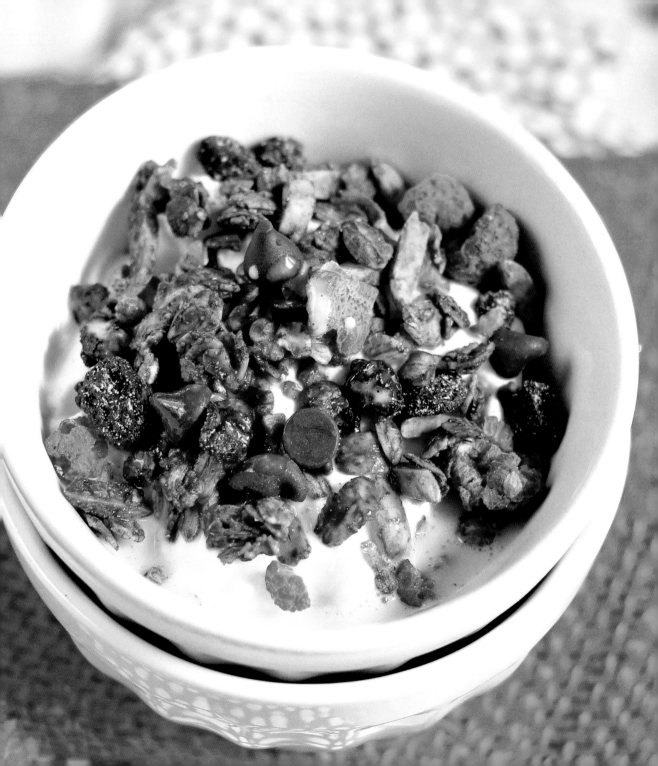

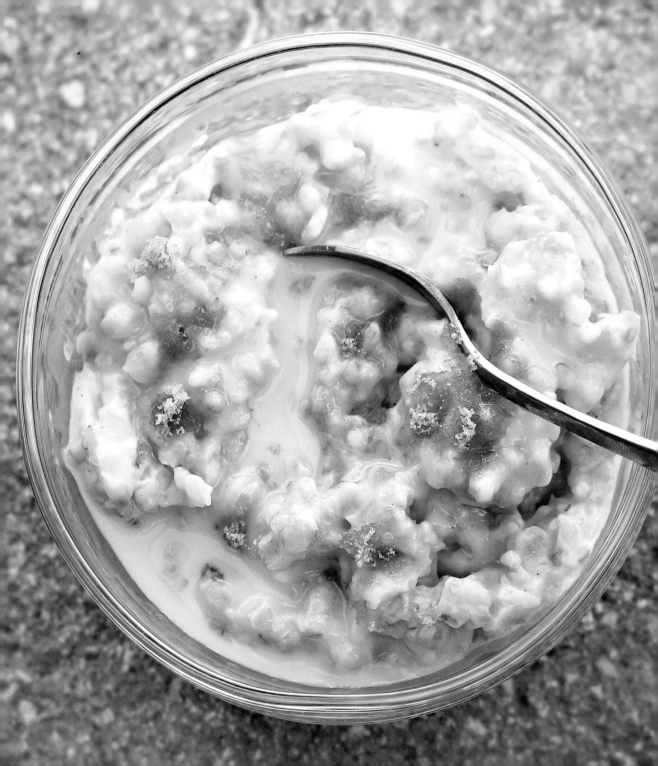

the creamiest oatmeal of your life

The name says it all. This is guaranteed to be the creamiest oatmeal you've ever tasted in your entire life. makes 4 to 6 servings

1 cup steel-cut oats

6 cups milk of choice

1/2 teaspoon salt

handful raisins, optional

2/3 cup pureed carrots or jarred carrot baby food

1 tablespoon pure vanilla extract

1/4 teaspoon pure stevia extract, or 1/2 cup sweetener of choice

7 to 8 tablespoons melted coconut butter or nut butter of choice

shredded coconut, optional

chopped walnuts, optional

In a medium pot, combine the oats, milk, salt, and raisins (if using). Bring to a boil over high heat. Turn the heat to low and continue to cook, uncovered and stirring occasionally, for 45 minutes, until the oatmeal thickens and becomes creamy.

Stir in the carrot puree, vanilla, and sweetener. Stir in the coconut butter until it is evenly mixed into the oatmeal. Stir in the shredded coconut and/or walnuts, if using. Refrigerate leftovers in a covered container for up to 3 days.

per serving

Calories	250	Fat	15 grams
Fiber	7 grams	Carbs	20 grams
Protein	7 grams	Weight Watchers PointsPlus Value	6

chocolate chip pumpkin bread

I've served this velvety pumpkin bread at many a breakfast gathering, and everyone is always shocked to discover that such a light and moist loaf contains no oil whatsoever! makes 1 loaf (12 servings)

1 cup canned pumpkin or pumpkin puree

$\frac{1}{2}$ cup milk of choice

2 tablespoons ground flax

1$\frac{1}{2}$ teaspoons pure vanilla extract

1 cup spelt flour or all-purpose flour *

$\frac{1}{4}$ cup plus 2 tablespoons xylitol or granulated sugar of choice

2 teaspoons cinnamon

$\frac{1}{2}$ teaspoon pumpkin pie spice

1 teaspoon baking powder

$\frac{1}{2}$ teaspoon baking soda

$\frac{1}{2}$ teaspoon salt

$\frac{1}{16}$ teaspoon pure stevia extract, or additional 2 tablespoons sugar of choice

$\frac{1}{2}$ cup mini chocolate chips

Preheat the oven to 350 degrees F. Grease an 8$\frac{1}{2}$x4$\frac{1}{2}$-inch loaf pan and set aside.

In a medium mixing bowl, whisk together the pumpkin, milk, flax, and vanilla. In a large mixing bowl, combine all remaining ingredients and stir very well.

Pour wet ingredients into dry and stir until just evenly combined. Transfer the batter to the prepared pan. Bake for 40 minutes, until the loaf has risen and a toothpick inserted into the middle comes out clean. Remove from the oven and allow to cool at least 15 minutes before slicing. Refrigerate leftovers in a covered container for up to 6 days.

per serving

Calories	80	Fat	2 grams
Fiber	2.5 grams	Carbs	14 grams
Protein	2.5 grams	Weight Watchers PointsPlus Value	2

*For a gluten-free version, substitute Bob's Red Mill gluten-free all-purpose baking flour for the flour, and add 1 teaspoon xanthan gum with the flour.

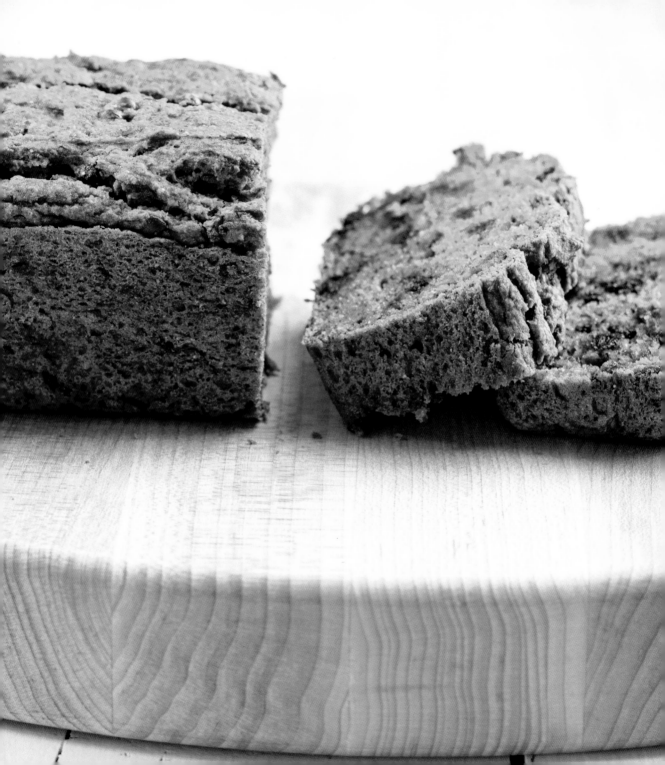

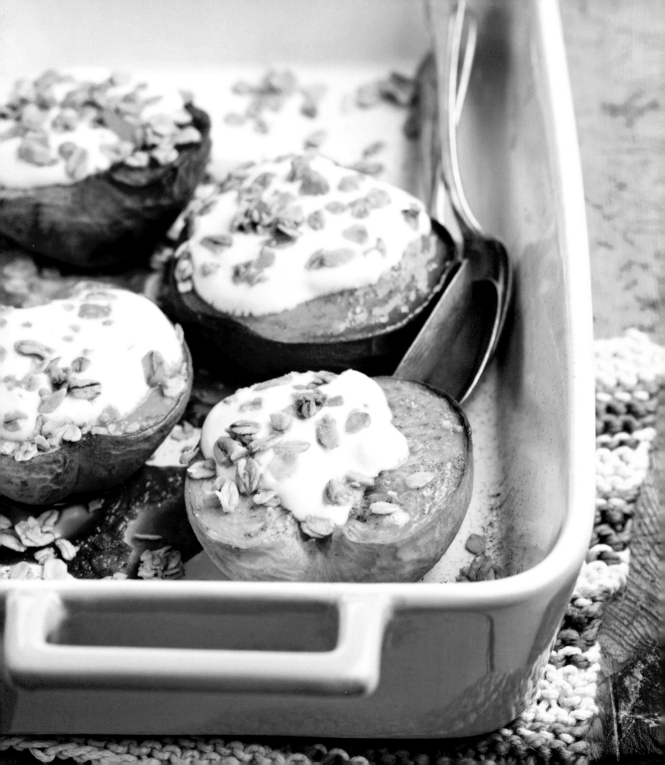

baked peaches with yogurt and granola

Fresh peaches are caramelized with pure maple syrup then topped with yogurt and granola for a healthy breakfast that tastes like peach pie. If you're feeling indulgent, feel free to replace the yogurt with Pure Bliss Vanilla Ice Cream (page 106) or your favorite ice cream.

makes 8 peach halves

4 ripe peaches, halved and pitted

2 tablespoons pure maple syrup or liquid sweetener of choice

1 teaspoon cinnamon

$^3/_4$ cup plain or vanilla yogurt of choice (I like WholeSoy or So Delicious cultured coconut milk)

$^1/_2$ cup Cinnamon Raisin Granola (page 79) or granola of choice

Preheat the oven to 375 degrees F. Line an 8-inch square pan with parchment paper.

Place the peach halves, cut side up, in the pan. Drizzle with the maple syrup, then evenly sprinkle the cinnamon on top. Bake for 60 minutes, until peaches are soft and the tops have browned. Remove from the oven and immediately top each peach half with 1$^1/_2$ tablespoons yogurt. Divide the granola evenly among the peaches.

per serving, with cinnamon raisin granola

Calories	65	Fat	3 grams
Fiber	3 grams	Carbs	18 grams
Protein	3 grams	Weight Watchers PointsPlus Value	2

chocoholic glazed doughnuts

Have you ever found yourself devouring a Krispy Kreme doughnut, licking the sticky-sweet glaze from your fingers and thinking, "Wow I really wish this glazed doughnut could be healthy"? Good news: Your wish has now been granted! Or maybe it was *my* wish…

makes 6 doughnuts

- $2/3$ cup milk of choice
- $2\frac{1}{2}$ tablespoons vegetable oil or melted coconut oil
- $1\frac{1}{2}$ teaspoons apple cider vinegar
- 1 teaspoon pure vanilla extract
- $3/4$ cup spelt flour or all-purpose flour*

- $1/3$ cup xylitol or granulated sugar of choice
- $1/16$ teaspoon pure stevia extract, or additional 2 tablespoons granulated sugar of choice
- $1/4$ cup cacao powder or unsweetened cocoa powder

- $1\frac{1}{2}$ teaspoons baking powder
- $1/4$ teaspoon salt
- Powdered Sugar Glaze (page 188); Chocolate Glaze 1 (opposite); or Chocolate Glaze 2 (opposite)

Preheat the oven to 350 degrees F. Lightly grease a doughnut pan and set aside.

In a small mixing bowl, whisk together the milk, oil, vinegar, and vanilla. Let sit at room temperature for at least 5 minutes. In a medium mixing bowl, combine all remaining ingredients except glaze and stir very well.

Pour wet ingredients into dry and stir until just evenly mixed. Portion the batter evenly among 6 doughnut molds so that each is about two-thirds full.

Bake for 13 minutes, until doughnuts have risen and a toothpick inserted into one comes out clean. Take out of the oven and allow to cool for 10 minutes before removing from the pan.

Frost doughnuts with glaze of choice. For a hard glaze, chill doughnuts directly after frosting, until the glaze hardens.

per doughnut, without glaze

Calories	120		Fat	6.5 grams
Fiber	3.5 grams		Carbs	15 grams
Protein	3 grams	Weight Watchers PointsPlus Value	3	

*For gluten-free doughnuts, substitute Bob's Red Mill gluten-free all-purpose baking flour for the flour, and add $\frac{1}{2}$ teaspoon xanthan gum with the flour.

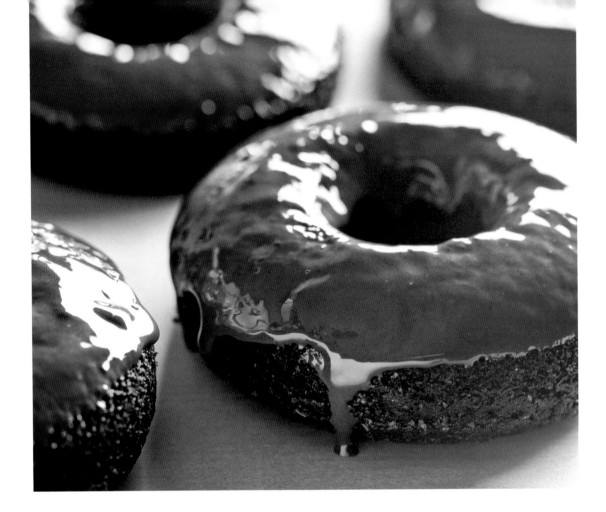

chocolate glaze 1

½ cup chocolate chips, melted

2 tablespoons vegetable oil or melted coconut oil

Combine all ingredients and stir.

chocolate glaze 2

¼ cup cacao powder or unsweetened cocoa powder

¼ cup virgin coconut oil, melted

1 tablespoon pure maple syrup or raw agave

Combine all ingredients and stir.

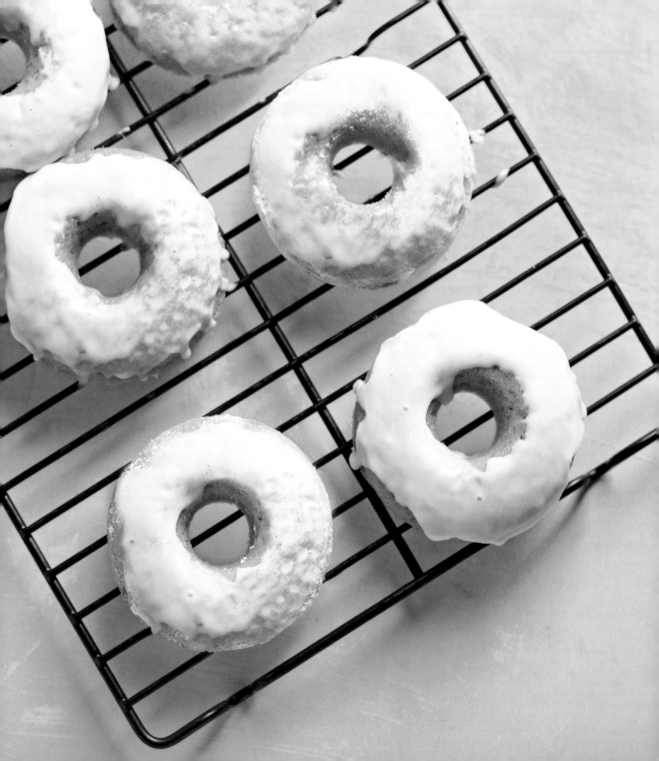

frosted lemon doughnuts

These bakery-style fluffy doughnuts have a lemon frosting that makes them completely irresistible! **makes 6 doughnuts**

- ½ cup milk of choice
- 2 teaspoons grated lemon zest
- 3 tablespoons lemon juice
- ¾ teaspoon pure vanilla extract
- 2½ tablespoons vegetable oil or melted coconut oil

- 1 cup spelt flour or all-purpose flour*
- ⅓ cup xylitol or granulated sugar of choice
- ¹⁄₁₆ teaspoon pure stevia extract, or additional 2 tablespoons sugar of choice

- 1½ teaspoons baking powder
- ¼ teaspoon salt
- Powdered Sugar Glaze (page 188), substituting lemon juice for the milk

Preheat the oven to 350 degrees F. Lightly grease a doughnut pan and set aside.

In a small mixing bowl, whisk together the milk, lemon zest, lemon juice, vanilla extract, and oil. Let sit at room temperature for at least 5 minutes. In a medium mixing bowl, combine all remaining ingredients and stir very well. Pour wet ingredients into dry and stir until just evenly mixed. Portion the batter evenly among 6 doughnut molds so that each is about two-thirds full.

Bake for 15 minutes, until doughnuts have risen and a toothpick inserted into one comes out clean. Take out of the oven and allow to cool for 10 minutes before removing from the pan.

Frost with glaze icing.

per glazed doughnut

Calories	130	Fat	6 grams
Fiber	3 grams	Carbs	17 grams
Protein	3 grams	Weight Watchers PointsPlus Value	3

*For gluten-free doughnuts, substitute Bob's Red Mill gluten-free all-purpose flour for the flour, and add ½ teaspoon xanthan gum with the flour.

sunday morning cinnamon rolls

You'd be hard-pressed to find another cinnamon roll with such a stellar nutritional profile as these low-calorie frosted breakfast pastries. With sweet cinnamon filling bursting into each and every bite, they can completely satisfy your craving for Cinnabon. No need to wait until Sunday... These family-friendly cinnamon rolls are good on weekdays too! makes 13 frosted cinnamon rolls

ROLLS
1 cup milk of choice

2 tablespoons sweetener of choice (excluding xylitol and stevia)

1 tablespoon active dry yeast

2½ cups plus 5 tablespoons spelt flour or all-purpose flour, divided

¼ cup granulated sugar of choice (I like Sucanat)

⅛ teaspoon pure stevia extract, or additional 3½ tablespoons granulated sugar of choice

2 tablespoons baking powder

2 teaspoons cinnamon

¾ teaspoon salt

¼ cup melted coconut oil or melted full-fat buttery spread (such as Earth Balance)

1 tablespoon pure vanilla extract

FILLING
1 cup applesauce

¼ cup granulated sugar of choice (I like Sucanat)

1 tablespoon cinnamon

dash salt

½ cup raisins, optional

GLAZE
1½ cups powdered sugar or Healthier Powdered Sugar (page 188)

1 tablespoon milk of choice

For the rolls: Lightly grease a large bowl and set aside. Using either a small pot on the stove or a medium bowl in the microwave, heat the milk until it is warm, but not boiling. If you have a candy thermometer, it should read 110 degrees F. Once the milk is warm, stir in the sweetener of choice, sprinkle the yeast on top, and set aside for 5 minutes, until the mixture begins to bubble. (If it does not bubble, either your yeast is no good or your milk was too hot or cold.)

In a large bowl, combine the 2½ cups flour, sugar of choice, stevia, baking powder, cinnamon, and salt. Stir very well. Stir the melted oil and vanilla into the milk mixture, then pour it into the large bowl of dry ingredients. Stir until a dough forms.

Form the dough into a ball. If necessary, add pinches of flour until the dough is firm enough to form a ball. Place in the greased large bowl. Cover loosely with a dry towel and set in a warm place for 20 minutes, until the dough has doubled in size. If your oven has a "bread proof" setting, this is a great option for a warm place to let your dough rise.

For the filling: In a medium bowl, stir together the applesauce, sugar of choice, cinnamon, salt, and raisins (if using). Set aside.

After the dough has risen, punch it to deflate. Knead the dough with your hands for 5 minutes, sprinkling the remaining 5 tablespoons flour over the dough as you knead so that it doesn't stick to your hands. On a lightly floured surface, roll out the dough into a very thin (about ¼-inch-thick) rectangle. Spread the filling evenly on top. Starting at a long side, carefully roll up the dough.

Lightly grease a 9x13-inch baking pan. Using a large, sharp knife, slice the rolled dough into 13 even rolls, wiping the knife after each cut. Don't worry if the filling oozes out a bit. Place the rolls in the prepared baking pan and return to the warm place to rise for 30 minutes.

Preheat the oven to 325 degrees F. Bake the cinnamon rolls for 20 minutes, until golden. Remove from the oven and allow to cool at least 10 minutes before adding the glaze.

For the glaze: Whisk the powdered sugar and milk together to form a thin glaze. If necessary, thin out the glaze by slowly adding more milk.

Using a spoon, drizzle the glaze evenly over the cinnamon rolls. Serve and enjoy!

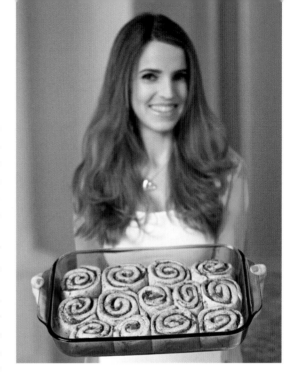

If you'd like hot cinnamon rolls first thing in the morning, follow all of the steps up to the baking step the night before. Cover the pan and refrigerate the rolls overnight. In the morning, place the pan in a cold oven and fill a separate shallow baking pan two-thirds full with boiling water. Set this shallow pan on the rack below the rolls. Close the oven and allow the rolls to rise for about 30 minutes. Remove both pans and preheat the oven to 325 degrees F. When it reaches this temperature, place only the cinnamon roll pan back in the oven and bake for 20 minutes, until golden.

per glazed roll

Calories	200	Fat	4.5 grams
Fiber	2.5 grams	Carbs	35 grams
Protein	3.5 grams	Weight Watchers PointsPlus Value	6

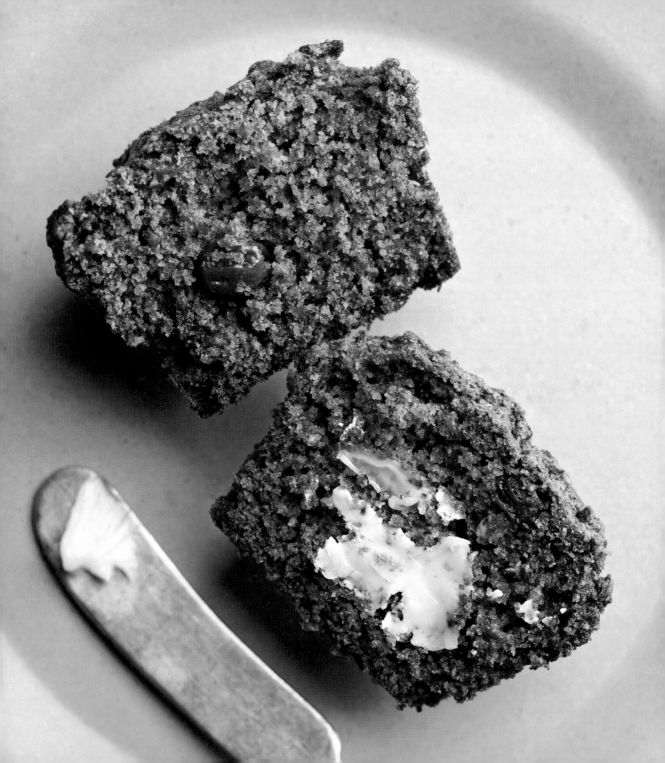

ironman muffins

Eating one of these heart-healthy muffins for breakfast will make you feel as strong as an Ironman…even if the only exercise you get all day is walking from the couch to the fridge. makes 12 muffins

2 cups bran flakes (I like Whole Foods 365 brand) or gluten-free alternative

1¼ cups milk of choice

¼ cup vegetable oil or melted coconut oil

2 tablespoons molasses

1 tablespoon ground flax

1¼ cups spelt flour, whole wheat pastry flour, or all-purpose flour*

½ cup granulated sugar of choice (I like Sucanat)

1 tablespoon baking powder

¼ teaspoon salt

⅔ cup raisins, optional

Preheat the oven to 400 degrees F. Grease a 12-cup muffin tin, or line with cupcake liners, and set aside.

In a large mixing bowl, combine the bran flakes and milk of choice. Set aside and allow to soak at room temperature for 30 to 40 minutes.

Whisk the oil, molasses, and flax into the bran flake mixture.

In a medium mixing bowl, combine all remaining ingredients and stir very well. Pour this dry mixture into the bowl with the bran flakes and stir until just evenly mixed. Portion the batter evenly among the muffin cups. Bake for 20 minutes, until lightly brown and fluffy and a toothpick inserted into the center of a muffin comes out clean. Take out of the oven and allow the muffins to cool for 10 minutes before removing from the tin.

per muffin

Calories	115	Fat	5 grams
Fiber	3 grams	Carbs	17 grams
Protein	3 grams	Weight Watchers PointsPlus Value	3

*For gluten-free muffins, substitute Bob's Red Mill gluten-free all-purpose baking flour for the flour, and add ¼ teaspoon xanthan gum with the flour.

raspberry orange corn muffins

Take out the fancy silverware and head for your kitchen. These muffins are the perfect excuse to host a fabulous Sunday brunch for all your closest friends. Even Martha Stewart would be impressed.

makes 12 muffins

1 cup milk of choice

3½ tablespoons vegetable oil or melted coconut oil

1 tablespoon grated orange zest

2 teaspoons apple cider vinegar

1 cup chopped raspberries

1 cup fine yellow cornmeal (whole grain or regular)

1 cup spelt flour or all-purpose flour *

⅓ cup xylitol or granulated sugar of choice

4 teaspoons baking powder

½ teaspoon salt

Preheat the oven to 400 degrees F. Grease a 12-cup muffin tin, or line with cupcake liners, and set aside.

In a medium mixing bowl, whisk together the milk, oil, zest, vinegar, and berries. Allow to sit at room temperature for at least 5 minutes. In a large mixing bowl, combine remaining ingredients and stir very well.

Pour wet ingredients into dry and stir until just evenly mixed. Portion the batter evenly among the muffin cups. Bake for 16 to 17 minutes, until muffins have risen, are lightly golden, and a toothpick inserted into the center of one comes out clean. Take out of the oven and allow to cool for 10 minutes before removing from the tin.

per muffin

Calories	115	Fat	4.5 grams
Fiber	3 grams	Carbs	16 grams
Protein	3 grams	Weight Watchers PointsPlus Value	3

*For gluten-free muffins, use certified-gluten-free cornmeal, substitute Bob's Red Mill gluten-free all-purpose baking flour for the flour, and add ¼ teaspoon xanthan gum with the flour.

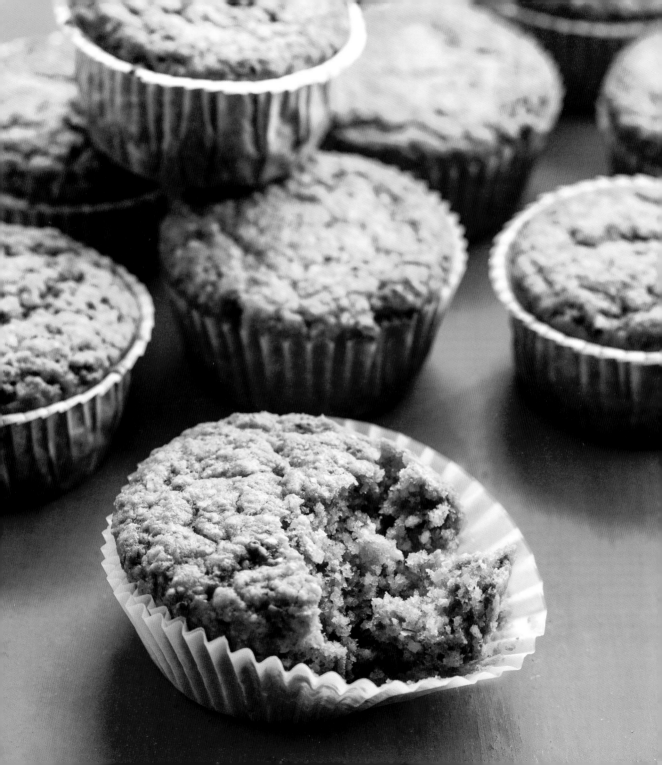

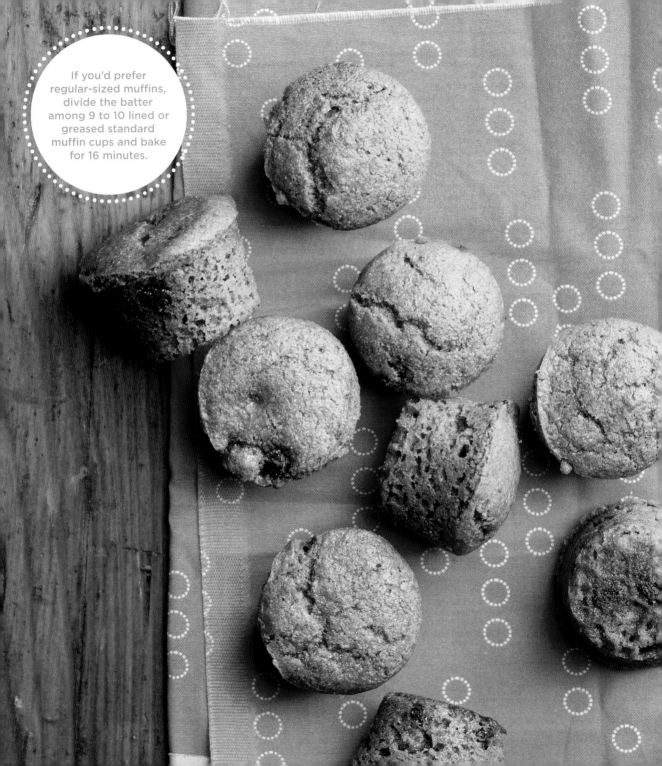

If you'd prefer regular-sized muffins, divide the batter among 9 to 10 lined or greased standard muffin cups and bake for 16 minutes.

cappuccino chocolate chip mini muffins

These mini muffins are addictive! You might find yourself actually *wanting* to get out of bed in the morning just to eat them. Since everyone else will have the same idea, you'd better get up early, before they're all gone! makes 24 to 28 mini muffins, or 9 to 10 standard muffins

- $3/4$ cup milk of choice
- 2 tablespoons vegetable oil or melted coconut oil
- 2 tablespoons plain yogurt of choice (I like WholeSoy or So Delicious cultured coconut milk)
- 2 teaspoons apple cider vinegar
- 2 teaspoons pure vanilla extract
- $1\frac{1}{4}$ cups spelt flour or all-purpose flour*
- $1/4$ cup xylitol or granulated sugar of choice
- $1/8$ teaspoon pure stevia extract, or additional 3 tablespoons granulated sugar of choice
- $2\frac{1}{4}$ teaspoons instant coffee granules
- $1\frac{1}{2}$ teaspoons baking powder
- $3/4$ teaspoon cinnamon
- $1/4$ teaspoon baking soda
- $3/8$ teaspoon salt
- $1/4$ cup mini chocolate chips

Preheat the oven to 400 degrees F. Grease a mini muffin tin, or line with mini cupcake liners, and set aside.

In a medium mixing bowl, whisk together the milk of choice, oil, yogurt, vinegar, and vanilla. Let sit at room temperature for at least 5 minutes. In a large mixing bowl, combine remaining ingredients and stir very well.

Pour wet ingredients into dry and stir until just evenly mixed. Portion the batter evenly among the muffin cups so that each is no more than two-thirds full. Bake for $8\frac{1}{2}$ minutes, until mini muffins have risen and a toothpick inserted into the center of one comes out clean.

Remove from the oven and allow to cool for 10 minutes before removing from the tin.

per mini muffin

Calories	30	Fat	1 gram
Fiber	1 gram	Carbs	5 grams
Protein	1 gram	Weight Watchers PointsPlus Value	1

*For gluten-free muffins, substitute Bob's Red Mill gluten-free all-purpose baking flour for the flour, and add $1/4$ teaspoon xanthan gum with the flour.

american as apple pie muffins

Soft, delicately spiced, and hot from the oven—if Grandma's famous apple pie were a muffin, it would taste like this. Try frosting them with Powdered Sugar Glaze (page 188) for Apple Fritter Muffins!

makes 12 muffins

1 cup milk of choice

1 cup peeled and finely diced apple

2½ tablespoons vegetable oil or melted coconut oil

1 tablespoon ground flax

1½ teaspoons pure vanilla extract

2 cups spelt flour or all-purpose flour*

½ cup xylitol or granulated sugar of choice

pinch pure stevia extract, or additional 1 tablespoon granulated sugar of choice

2 teaspoons baking powder

½ teaspoon cinnamon

½ teaspoon plus ⅛ teaspoon salt

½ cup raisins, optional

Preheat the oven to 350 degrees F. Grease a 12-cup muffin tin, or line with cupcake liners, and set aside.

In a medium mixing bowl, whisk together the milk, apple, oil, flax, and vanilla. Let sit at room temperature for at least 5 minutes. In a large mixing bowl, combine all remaining ingredients and stir very well.

Pour wet ingredients into dry and stir until just evenly mixed. Portion the batter evenly among the muffin cups. Bake for 20 minutes, until muffins have risen and are lightly golden and a toothpick inserted into the center of one comes out clean. Remove from the oven and allow to cool for 10 minutes before removing from the tin.

per muffin

Calories	105	Fat	3.5 grams
Fiber	3 grams	Carbs	17.5 grams
Protein	3 grams	Weight Watchers PointsPlus Value	3

*For gluten-free muffins, substitute Bob's Red Mill gluten-free all-purpose baking flour for the flour, and add ½ teaspoon xanthan gum with the flour.

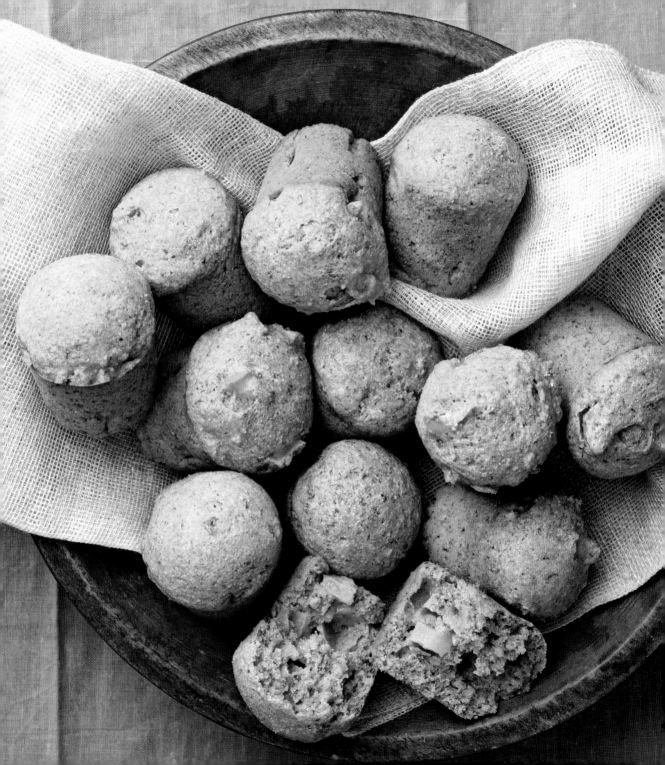

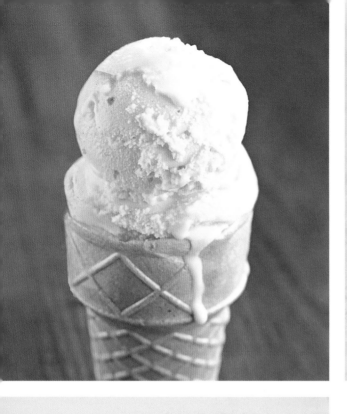
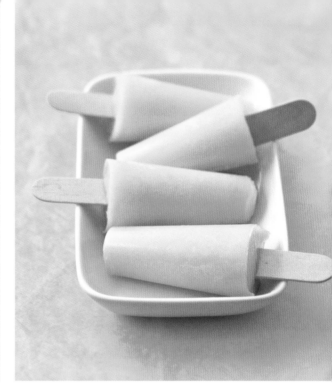
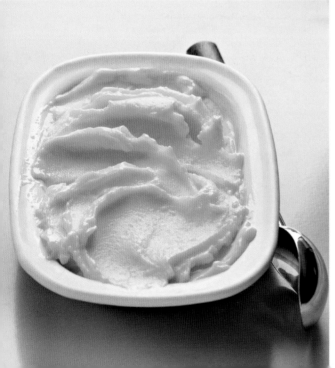
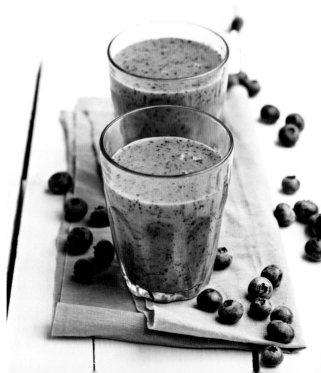

4

ice cream,
milkshakes
& smoothies

coffee chocolate chip ice cream

After giving up dairy 12 years ago, I missed ice cream like crazy and found myself disappointed again and again with the non-dairy options on the market. Craving the indulgently rich and smooth creaminess of Häagen-Dazs and Ben & Jerry's, I set out to make a homemade version that would rival the taste and texture of those classic brands. It took me over a year to get the recipe just right, but the result was definitely worth the wait! makes 3 to 4 servings

---

1 cup raw cashews or macadamia nuts

1¼ cups milk of choice

3 tablespoons xylitol, pure maple syrup, or granulated sugar of choice

¹⁄₁₆ teaspoon pure stevia extract, or additional 2 tablespoons sweetener of choice

1½ teaspoons instant coffee granules

1½ teaspoons pure vanilla extract

⅛ teaspoon plus ¹⁄₁₆ teaspoon salt

mini chocolate chips or homemade chocolate chips (see page 198), amount optional

---

In a small bowl, cover the nuts with water. Set aside to soak at room temperature for 6 to 8 hours. Drain completely and pat dry.

Combine soaked nuts and all remaining ingredients except the chocolate chips in a blender and blend until all the nut pieces have disappeared and the mixture is completely smooth.

Follow one of the ice cream making methods below, or pour the mixture into popsicle molds and freeze to make popsicles.

Vitamix method: Pour the mixture into two ice-cube trays and freeze until solid. Once frozen, pop out the cubes into your Vitamix by pushing a knife down one side of each section of the trays. Blend, using the tamper, until completely smooth with a soft-serve texture. Stir in the chocolate chips, if desired. Scoop out into individual bowls, using an ice cream scoop for authentic presentation. Serve immediately, or freeze each bowl up to 1 hour for a thicker consistency and texture.

Ice cream maker method: Pour the blended mixture into a large container. Freeze for 30 minutes or refrigerate for at least 4 hours. Pour chilled mixture into the ice cream maker and follow the manufacturer's instructions. Once a smooth texture has been reached, turn off the machine and stir in the chocolate chips, if desired. Scoop out into individual bowls, using an ice cream scoop for authentic presentation. Serve immediately as soft serve, or freeze each bowl up to an hour for a thicker consistency and texture.

Food processor method: Pour the mixture into two ice-cube trays and freeze until solid. Once frozen, pop out the cubes into your food processor by pushing a knife down one side of each section of the trays. Allow to thaw just long enough for your food processor to be able to handle the ice cubes without overheating. Process on high, stopping occasionally to scrape down the sides. Stir in the chocolate chips, if desired. Scoop out into individual bowls, using an ice cream scoop for authentic presentation. Serve immediately, or freeze

each bowl up to 1 hour for a thicker consistency and texture. Note: Using a food processor will yield more of a soft-serve consistency than the other two methods listed here.

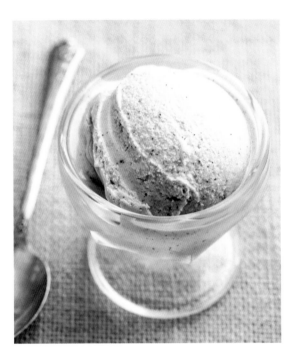

Storing Leftovers

Due to the lack of chemicals and stabilizers, as well as the lower sugar content, the ice cream recipes in this book will have the creamiest texture the day they are made. However, the ice cream will keep in the freezer for up to a month. It is best to portion out the ice cream, covering each individual bowl, before freezing. Remove each portion from the freezer 20 to 25 minutes before serving so it can thaw back into a smooth ice cream.

per ½-cup serving

Calories	180	Fat	14 grams
Fiber	1.5 grams	Carbs	12 grams
Protein	5 grams	Weight Watchers PointsPlus Value	6

pure bliss vanilla ice cream

Four ingredients magically come together for a dreamy homemade ice cream without any cream or eggs! Serve on top of your favorite pie, or scoop the ice cream into a bowl or cone and cover with sliced bananas, strawberries, and chocolate syrup. **makes 3 to 4 servings**

2 cups milk of choice (see note on opposite page)

$1/8$ heaping teaspoon pure stevia extract, or

$1/3$ cup sweetener of choice

$1^1/2$ teaspoons pure vanilla extract

$1/8$ teaspoon salt

In a medium mixing bowl, whisk together the ingredients. Follow one of the ice cream making methods below, or pour the mixture into popsicle molds and freeze to make popsicles.

Vitamix method: Pour the mixture into two ice-cube trays and freeze until solid. Once frozen, pop out the cubes into your Vitamix by pushing a knife down one side of each section of the trays. Blend, using the tamper, until completely smooth with a soft-serve texture. Serve immediately as soft serve, or transfer to a covered container and freeze up to an hour for firmer texture. Scoop out with an ice cream scoop for authentic presentation.

Ice cream maker method: Pour the mixture into a large container. Freeze for 30 minutes or refrigerate for at least 4 hours. Pour chilled mixture into the ice cream maker and follow the manufacturer's instructions. Once a smooth texture has been reached, scoop out into individual bowls, using an ice cream scoop for authentic presentation. Serve immediately as soft serve, or freeze each bowl up to an hour for a thicker consistency and texture.

Food processor method: Pour the mixture into two ice-cube trays and freeze until solid. Once frozen, pop out the cubes into your food processor by pushing a knife down one side of each section of the tray. Allow to thaw just long enough for your food processor to be able to handle the ice cubes without overheating. Process on high, stopping occasionally to scrape down the sides. Scoop out into individual bowls, using an ice cream scoop for authentic presentation. Serve immediately, or freeze each bowl up to 1 hour for a thicker consistency and texture. Note: Using a food processor will yield more of a soft-serve consistency than the other two methods listed on this page.

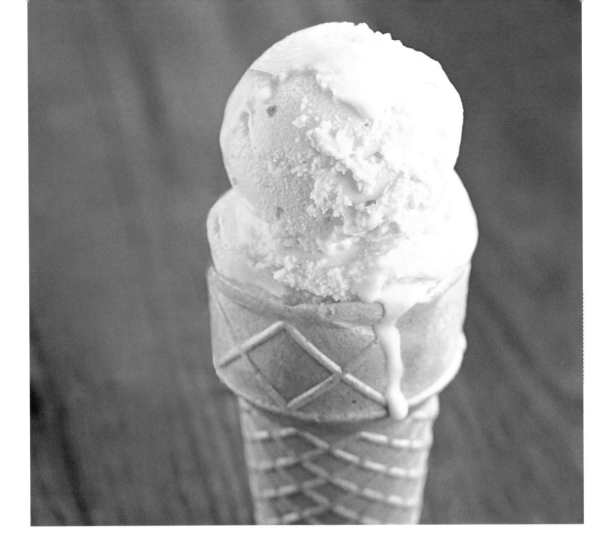

For the best ice cream–like taste and texture in this recipe use either Cashew Cream (see page 135) or full-fat canned coconut milk as your milk of choice. It will still be delicious if you use a lower-fat milk, such as almond or soy milk, but the texture will be less creamy.

per ½-cup serving

Calories	15	Fat	1 gram
Fiber	0 grams	Carbs	.5 gram
Protein	.5 gram	Weight Watchers PointsPlus Value	0

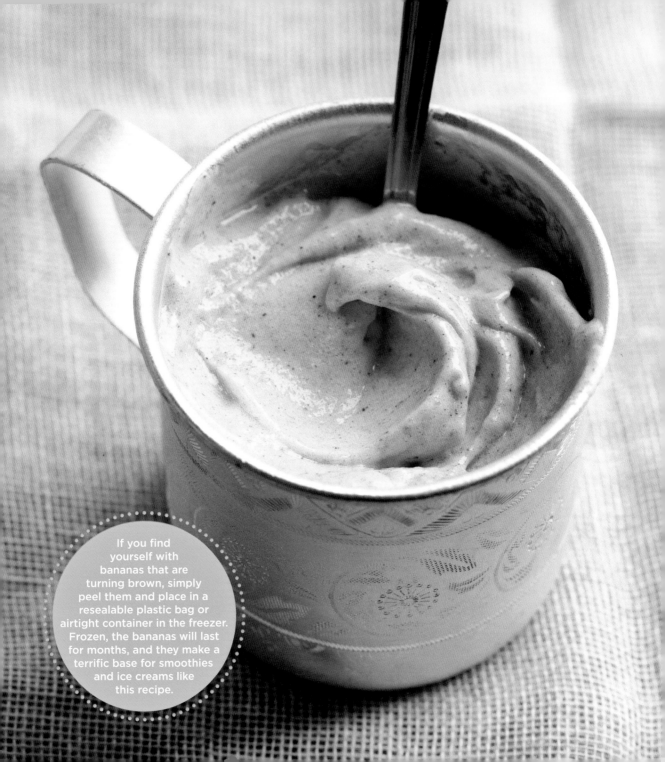

If you find yourself with bananas that are turning brown, simply peel them and place in a resealable plastic bag or airtight container in the freezer. Frozen, the bananas will last for months, and they make a terrific base for smoothies and ice creams like this recipe.

chai banana soft serve

Something magical happens when you swirl frozen bananas in a blender. The fruit suddenly turns into a smooth confection with almost the exact texture of soft-serve ice cream! Although this particular recipe is quite spicy—and therefore meant for hard-core chai lovers—you can easily omit the spices for a plain banana soft serve. Or let your creativity shine by adding any mix-ins your heart desires. Chocolate chips and peanut butter? Strawberries and vanilla bean paste? Peppermint extract and cocoa powder? The sky is definitely *not* the limit. makes 3 to 4 servings

4 frozen, peeled, and over-ripe bananas, broken into large pieces

$3/4$ teaspoon ground ginger

$3/4$ teaspoon cinnamon

$1/2$ teaspoon pure vanilla extract

$1/8$ teaspoon nutmeg

$1/8$ teaspoon ground cloves

$1/8$ teaspoon ground cardamom

pinch salt

pinch black pepper, optional

$1/4$ cup almond butter or melted coconut butter, optional

2 tablespoons milk of choice, plus 1 additional tablespoon if needed for smooth blending

Blend all ingredients in a food processor, blender, or Vitamix until a smooth and creamy texture is reached. Add the extra tablespoon milk of choice if needed for smooth blending. Serve immediately.

per $1/2$-cup serving

Calories	105	Fat	0 grams
Fiber	3.5 grams	Carbs	26.5 grams
Protein	1.5 grams	Weight Watchers PointsPlus Value	3

pistachio ice cream

This healthy version of the ice cream parlor classic has the same flavor and creaminess of traditional pistachio ice cream but none of the artificial additives or colorings. makes 3 to 4 servings

1 cup shelled unsalted raw pistachios

$1\frac{1}{4}$ cups milk of choice

3 tablespoons xylitol, pure maple syrup, or granulated sugar of choice

$\frac{1}{16}$ teaspoon pure stevia extract, or additional 2 tablespoons sweetener of choice

$1\frac{1}{2}$ teaspoons pure vanilla extract

$\frac{1}{8}$ teaspoon plus $\frac{1}{16}$ teaspoon salt

In a small bowl, cover the pistachios with water. Set aside to soak at room temperature for 6 to 8 hours. Drain completely and pat dry.

Combine the soaked nuts and all remaining ingredients in a blender and blend until all pistachio pieces have disappeared and the mixture is completely smooth. Follow one of the ice cream making methods below, or pour the mixture into popsicle molds and freeze to make popsicles.

Vitamix method: Pour the mixture into two ice-cube trays and freeze until solid. Once frozen, pop out the cubes into your Vitamix by pushing a knife down one side of each section. Blend, using the tamper, until completely smooth with a soft-serve texture. Scoop out into individual bowls, using an ice cream scoop for authentic presentation. Serve immediately as soft serve, or cover and freeze each bowl up to 1 hour for a thicker consistency and texture.

Ice cream maker method: Pour the blended mixture into a large container and freeze for 30 minutes or refrigerate for at least 4 hours. Pour chilled mixture into the ice cream maker and follow the manufacturer's instructions. Once the desired texture has been reached, scoop out into individual bowls, using an ice cream scoop for authentic presentation. Serve immediately, or cover and freeze each bowl up to 1 hour for a thicker consistency and texture.

Food processor method: Pour the mixture into two ice-cube trays and freeze until solid. Once frozen, pop out the cubes into your food processor by pushing a knife down one side of each section of the trays. Allow to thaw just long enough for your food processor to be able to handle the ice cubes without overheating. Process on high, stopping occasionally to scrape down the sides. Scoop out into individual bowls, using an ice cream scoop for

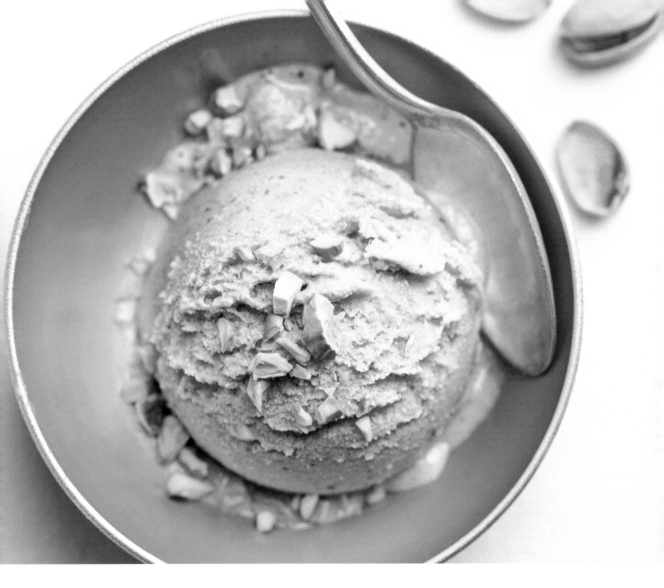

authentic presentation. Serve immediately, or cover and freeze each bowl up to 1 hour for a thicker consistency and texture. Note: Using a food processor will yield more of a soft-serve consistency than the other two methods listed here.

Calories	175		Fat	13 grams
Fiber	1.5 grams		Carbs	11 grams
Protein	5 grams		Weight Watchers PointsPlus Value	5

chocolate peanut butter cup ice cream

To take this recipe over the top, stir in some bite-sized pieces of Secretly Healthy Brownies (page 38). **makes 3 to 4 servings**

1½ cups milk of choice

⅓ cup peanut butter

3 tablespoons cacao powder or unsweetened cocoa powder

⅛ teaspoon pure stevia extract, or ¼ cup sweetener of choice

½ teaspoon pure vanilla extract

⅛ teaspoon salt

Combine all ingredients in a blender, or stir very well by hand, until completely smooth. Follow one of the ice cream making methods below, or pour the mixture into popsicle molds and freeze to make popsicles.

Vitamix method: Pour the mixture into two ice-cube trays and freeze until solid. Once frozen, pop out the ice cubes into your Vitamix by pushing a knife down one side of each section of the trays. Blend, using the tamper, until completely smooth with a soft-serve texture. Scoop out into individual bowls, using an ice cream scoop for authentic presentation. Serve immediately as soft serve, or freeze each bowl up to 1 hour for a thicker consistency and texture.

Ice cream maker method: Pour the mixture into a large container and freeze for 30 minutes or refrigerate for at least 4 hours. Pour chilled mixture into an ice cream maker and churn according to manufacturer's directions. Serve immediately as soft serve, or transfer to an airtight container and freeze up to 1 hour for firmer texture.

Food processor method: Pour the mixture into two ice-cube trays and freeze until solid. Once frozen, pop out the cubes into your food processor by pushing a knife down one side of each section of the trays. Allow to thaw just long enough for your food processor to be able to handle the ice cubes without overheating. Process on high, stopping occasionally to scrape down the sides. Scoop out into individual bowls, using an ice cream scoop for authentic presentation. Serve immediately, or freeze each bowl up to 1 hour for a thicker consistency and texture. Note: Using a food processor will yield more of a soft-serve consistency than the other two methods listed on this page.

per ½-cup serving

Calories	180		Fat	15 grams
Fiber	3.5 grams		Carbs	8.5 grams
Protein	8.5 grams	Weight Watchers PointsPlus Value	5

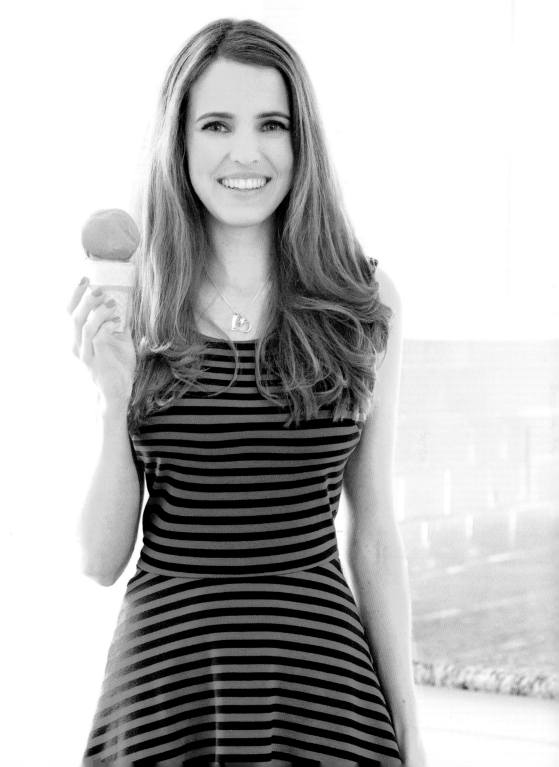

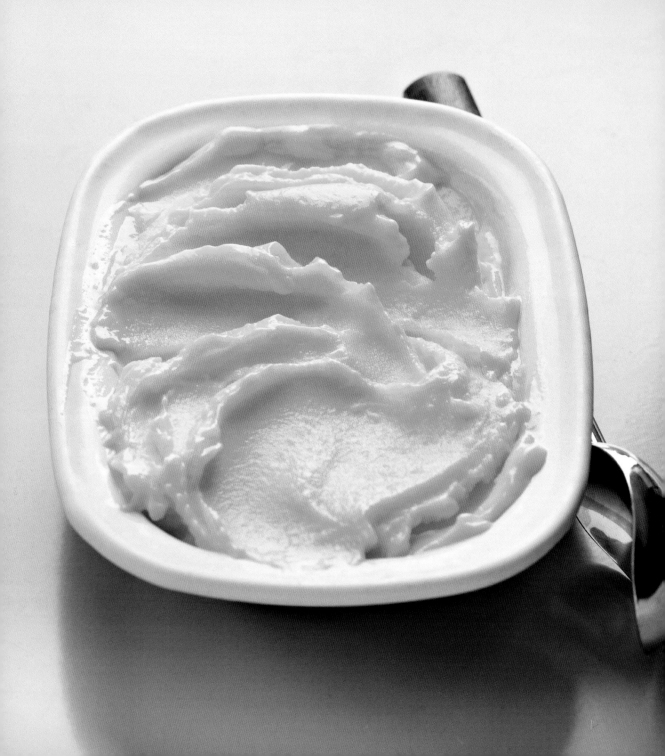

sunrise mango sherbet

Who knew something so simple could taste so divine?

4 cups frozen mango slices

½ cup milk of choice

pinch pure stevia extract, or 1½ tablespoons sweetener of choice

Blend all ingredients in a food processor, blender, or Vitamix until a smooth and creamy texture is reached. Serve as soft serve, or transfer to an airtight container and freeze for up to 1 hour.

Store any leftovers in an airtight container for up to a month; thaw 15 to 20 minutes before serving.

per ½-cup serving

Calories	110	Fat	.5 gram
Fiber	3 grams	Carbs	27 grams
Protein	1 gram	Weight Watchers PointsPlus Value	free food

peanut butter pudding pops

This simple summer treat will make you feel like a kid again—running around in the sunshine, riding your bike through the neighborhood streets, then cooling off with a creamy homemade pudding pop. Enjoy one after a strenuous workout or as an escape from the relentless summer heat. makes 8 pops, depending on the size of your popsicle molds

2 large, over-ripe bananas

1½ cups milk of choice

½ cup peanut butter or allergy-friendly alternative (if unsalted, add a pinch more salt)

⅛ teaspoon pure stevia extract, or ¼ cup granulated sweetener of choice (see note on opposite page)

⅛ teaspoon salt

Blend all ingredients in a food processor, blender, or Vitamix until a smooth and creamy texture is reached. Pour into popsicle molds. If you don't have popsicle molds, simply pour the mixture into mini Dixie cups. Freeze for about 20 minutes, then stick a small spoon or a popsicle stick (which can be purchased at craft stores) into each cup. Place pops back in the freezer and freeze until frozen solid.

per popsicle, based on 8

Calories	130	Fat	8.5 grams
Fiber	2.5 grams	Carbs	11 grams
Protein	5 grams	Weight Watchers PointsPlus Value	4

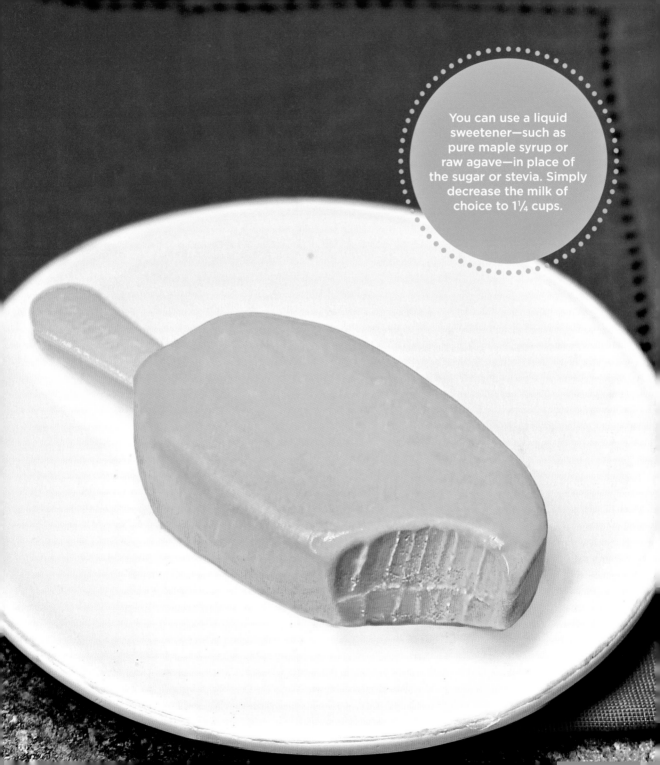

You can use a liquid sweetener—such as pure maple syrup or raw agave—in place of the sugar or stevia. Simply decrease the milk of choice to 1¼ cups.

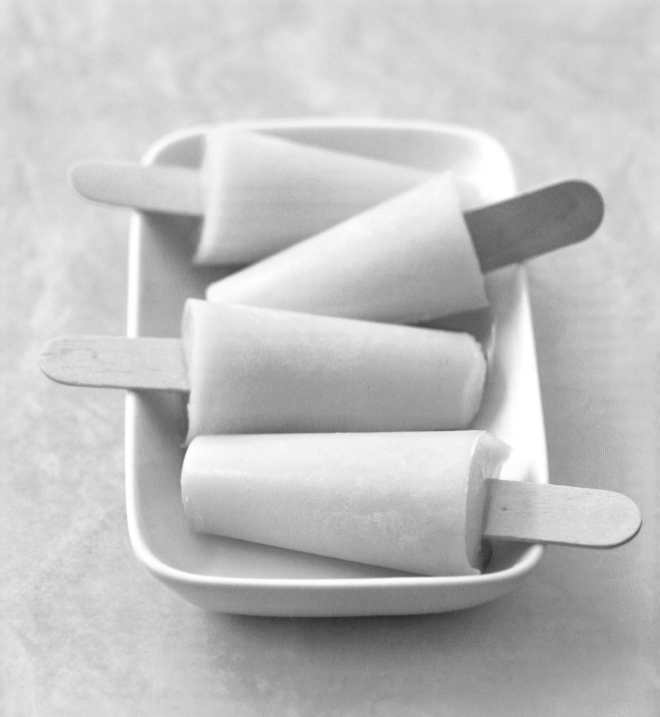

tropical pineapple popsicles

Eating these popsicles is the next-best thing to being on a beach in Hawaii. For the full tropical experience, I highly recommend using canned coconut milk as your milk of choice.

makes 8, depending on the size of your popsicle molds

2 cups frozen pineapple, or 1 (20-ounce) can pineapple chunks, drained

1/4 cup milk of choice

2 teaspoons lemon juice

pinch salt

1/16 teaspoon pure stevia extract, or 2 tablespoons sweetener of choice

Blend all ingredients in a food processor, blender, or Vitamix until a smooth and creamy texture is reached. Pour into popsicle molds. If you don't have popsicle molds, simply pour the mixture into mini Dixie cups. Freeze for about 20 minutes, then stick a small spoon or a popsicle stick (which can be purchased at craft stores) into each cup. Place pops back in the freezer and freeze until frozen solid.

per popsicle, based on 8

Calories	35	Fat	0 grams
Fiber	1 gram	Carbs	9 grams
Protein	0 grams	Weight Watchers PointsPlus Value	1

frozen hot chocolate

A recipe inspired by the cult classic dessert from New York's famous Serendipity restaurant. If you've never tried frozen hot chocolate, you are in for an enchanting experience. makes 1 large or 2 smaller servings

½ cup full-fat canned coconut milk or Cashew Cream (page 135)

½ cup milk of choice

2 tablespoons cacao powder or unsweetened cocoa powder

⅟₁₆ teaspoon pure stevia extract, or 2 tablespoons sweetener of choice

pinch salt

Stovetop method: Combine all ingredients in a small saucepan. Place over medium heat and whisk for 3 to 5 minutes, until the cacao powder is completely dissolved.

Microwave method: Combine all ingredients in a medium microwave-safe bowl and microwave in three to four 30-second intervals, stirring after each interval, until the cacao powder is completely dissolved.

Allow the mixture to cool at least 10 minutes, then pour into an ice-cube tray and freeze until completely frozen. Once frozen, place the chocolate ice cubes in a food processor, blender, or Vitamix and blend until a smooth and creamy texture is reached. If your blender is not as powerful as a Vitamix, you may need to thaw the cubes just long enough for your blender to handle them without overheating. Top with Coconut Whipped Cream (page 183) if desired.

per ½ of the recipe

Calories	155	Fat	15 grams
Fiber	4 grams	Carbs	6.5 grams
Protein	3 grams	Weight Watchers PointsPlus Value	5

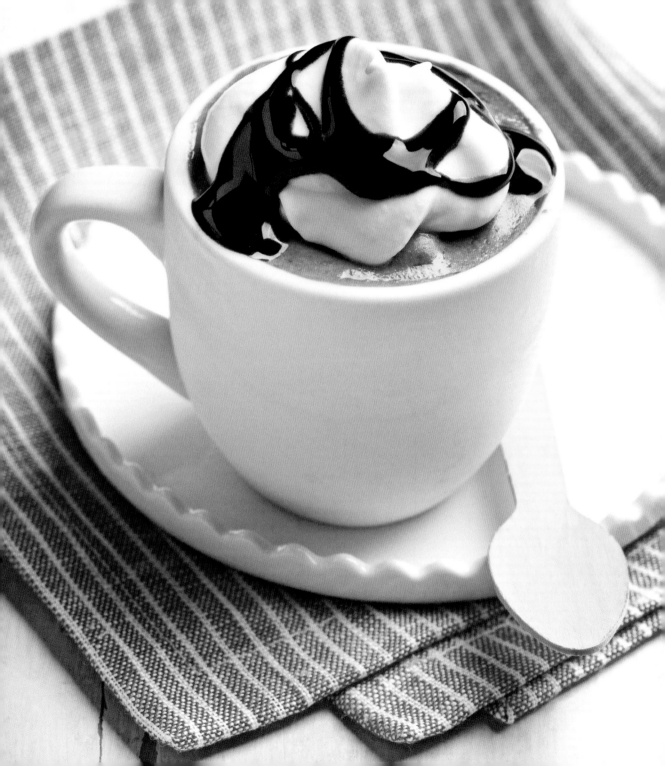

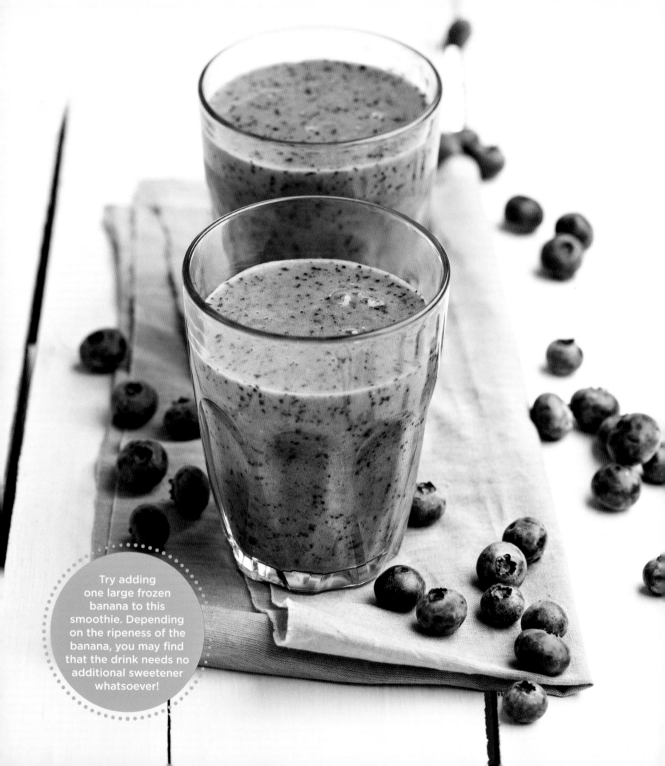

Try adding one large frozen banana to this smoothie. Depending on the ripeness of the banana, you may find that the drink needs no additional sweetener whatsoever!

the blueberry beauty queen

Fitting the recommended eight or more servings of fruits and veggies in each day can be a daunting and frustrating task. Thankfully, you can whip up a smoothie almost instantly, packing multiple fruit and veggie servings into a single glass. With an energizing antioxidant boost, just one serving of this vibrantly beautiful berry smoothie gets you almost halfway to your daily recommended total! makes 1 serving

1 large orange, peeled and seeded

1 cup frozen blueberries

½ cup milk of choice

¼ teaspoon pure vanilla extract

tiny pinch salt

1 scoop vanilla protein powder of choice, optional

sweetener of choice, to taste (see note on opposite page)

Blend all ingredients together in a blender, Magic Bullet, or Vitamix until completely smooth.

per serving

Calories	180	Fat	1.5 grams
Fiber	9 grams	Carbs	40 grams
Protein	3.5 grams	Weight Watchers PointsPlus Value	4

the mint chocolate chip milkshake

This minty milkshake is quite possibly one of the easiest and most delicious healthy recipes you will ever find. Thanks to the spinach and banana, it is packed with nutrition while simultaneously tasting like a thick ice cream shake. As soon as I finish drinking one, I almost always find myself right back in the kitchen for another! makes 1 serving

1 frozen, peeled, and over-ripe very large banana, cut into large pieces (see note on opposite page)

1 cup milk of choice

1/4 teaspoon pure peppermint extract, or more if desired

pinch salt

1/4 cup frozen spinach, optional (for color and added nutrition)

1 scoop vanilla protein powder of choice, optional

sweetener of choice, to taste

chocolate chips or homemade chocolate chips (see page 198) or cacao nibs, optional for garnish

Blend all ingredients except the garnishes in a blender, Magic Bullet, or Vitamix until completely smooth. Garnish as desired.

If you can't get on board with the greens-in-smoothies thing, it is completely fine to leave out the spinach. If you still would like a natural green hue, try adding a pinch of spirulina powder, a superfood powder abundant with vitamins and minerals. Look for spirulina in health food stores or online.

per serving

Calories	150	Fat	2.5 grams
Fiber	5.5 grams	Carbs	32 grams
Protein	2.5 grams	Weight Watchers PointsPlus Value	4

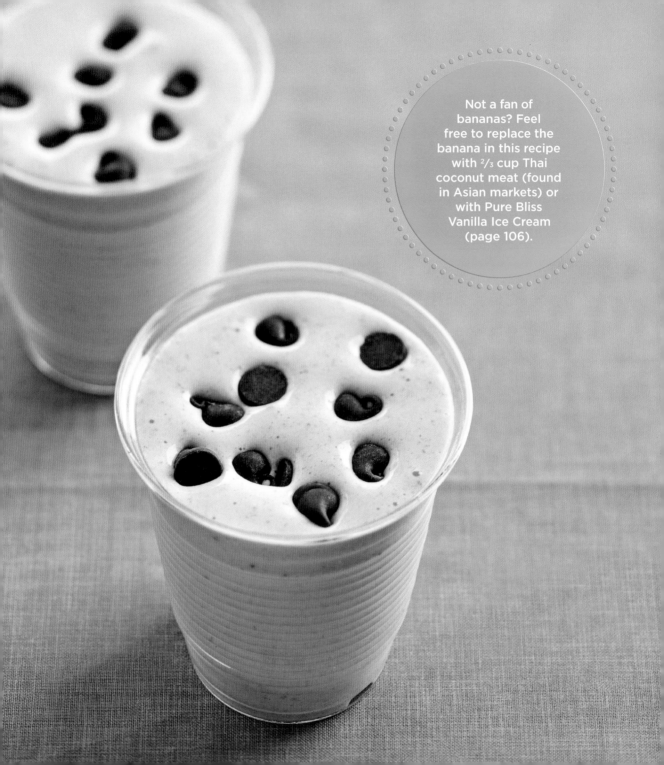

Not a fan of bananas? Feel free to replace the banana in this recipe with ⅔ cup Thai coconut meat (found in Asian markets) or with Pure Bliss Vanilla Ice Cream (page 106).

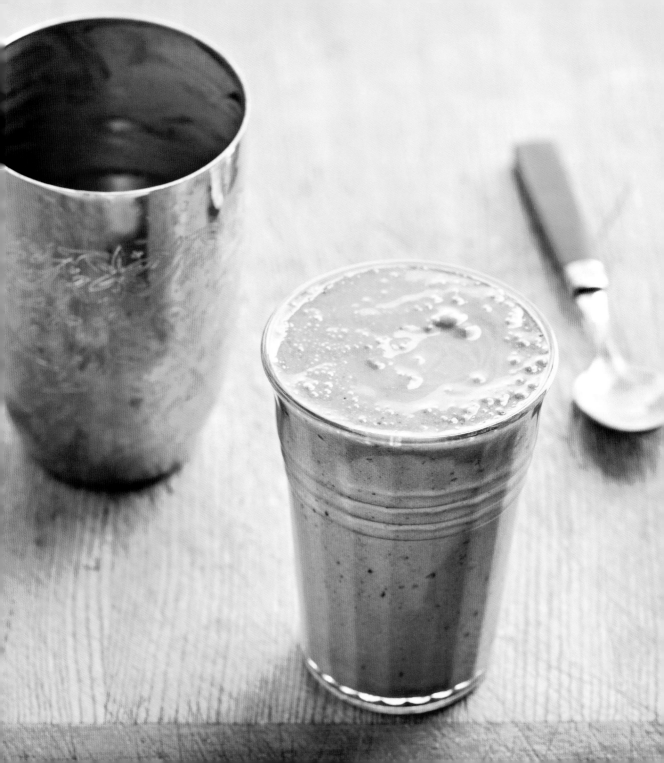

the chocolate-covered cherry

Cherries are an outstanding post-workout choice. Full of vitamins, they help to reduce inflammation, send much-needed oxygen to muscles, and speed up the recovery process. With this thick chocolate smoothie, you're also getting antioxidants from the cacao powder and probiotics from the yogurt. And it tastes like a chocolate-covered cherry! makes 1 serving

$^2/_3$ cup frozen cherries

$^1/_2$ cup plain yogurt of choice (I like WholeSoy)

$^1/_3$ cup milk of choice

1 tablespoon cacao powder or unsweetened cocoa powder

pinch salt

handful raw spinach, optional

2 tablespoons almond butter, optional

1 tablespoon chocolate or vanilla protein powder of choice, optional

sweetener of choice, to taste

Blend all ingredients together in a blender, Magic Bullet, or Vitamix until completely smooth.

per serving

Calories	230	Fat	3 grams
Fiber	5 grams	Carbs	49 grams
Protein	6 grams	Weight Watchers PointsPlus Value	3

the bananaccino

Forget about that fancy coffee shop down the street. This homemade frozen coffee drink offers an instant pick-me-up any time you're feeling sluggish, and the best part is there's no need to get out of your pajamas!

makes 1 serving

1 frozen, peeled, and over-ripe banana, broken into large pieces

1 cup milk of choice

1 teaspoon instant coffee granules, regular or decaf

½ teaspoon pure vanilla extract

¼ teaspoon cinnamon

1/16 teaspoon salt

1 scoop protein powder of choice, optional

sweetener of choice, to taste

Blend all ingredients together in a blender, Magic Bullet, or Vitamix until completely smooth.

per serving

Calories	135	Fat	2.5 grams
Fiber	5 grams	Carbs	27.5 grams
Protein	2.5 grams	Weight Watchers PointsPlus Value	3

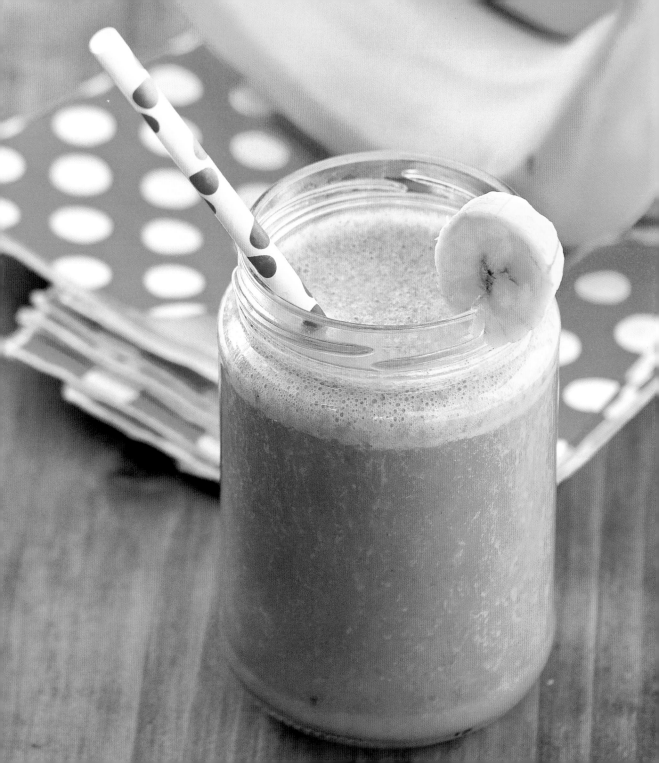

the chocolate mudslide

One of my top five favorite recipes in the book! The avocado makes this lavish milkshake so thick and creamy you'll swear it must be full of unhealthy fat and calories. But surprisingly, it's not at all!

makes 1 serving

$\frac{1}{3}$ of a large, ripe avocado (about $\frac{1}{4}$ cup mashed)

$\frac{3}{4}$ cup milk of choice

$1\frac{1}{2}$ tablespoons cacao powder or unsweetened cocoa powder

1 tablespoon liquid sweetener of choice (I like pure maple syrup)

pinch pure stevia extract, or additional $1\frac{1}{2}$ teaspoons liquid sweetener of choice

1 teaspoon pure vanilla extract

$\frac{1}{16}$ teaspoon salt

2 ice cubes

Blend all ingredients together in a blender, Magic Bullet, or Vitamix until completely smooth.

per serving

Calories	155	Fat	8.5 grams
Fiber	5.5 grams	Carbs	20 grams
Protein	3 grams	Weight Watchers PointsPlus Value	4

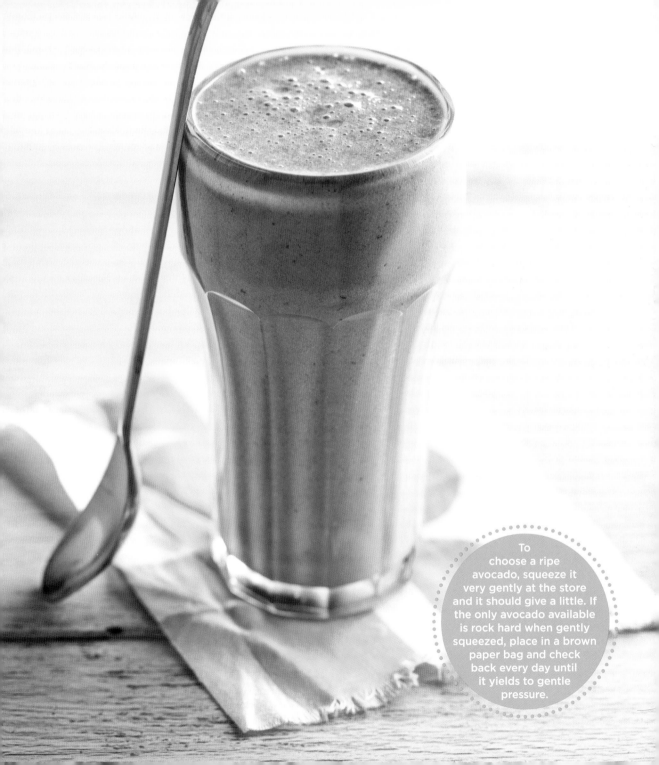

To choose a ripe avocado, squeeze it very gently at the store and it should give a little. If the only avocado available is rock hard when gently squeezed, place in a brown paper bag and check back every day until it yields to gentle pressure.

the passionate peach

With an invigorating blend of fresh strawberries, coconut water, and sweet peaches, this smoothie is like summer in a glass.

makes 1 large serving

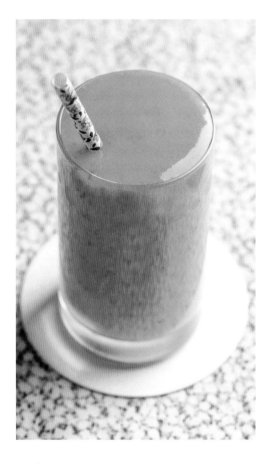

1 ripe peach, pitted and sliced

5 strawberries, stems removed

$^2/_3$ cup chilled coconut water (I highly

recommend Harmless Harvest brand or fresh coconut water straight from the coconut)

sweetener of choice, to taste

Blend all ingredients together in a blender, Magic Bullet, or Vitamix until completely smooth.

per serving

Calories	85	Fat	.5 gram
Fiber	8.5 grams	Carbs	20 grams
Protein	2.5 grams	Weight Watchers PointsPlus Value	2

You can either remove the peach peel or leave it intact. I normally choose to wash the fruit and leave the peel intact, especially if the peach is organic. The outer skin of the peach contains fiber and antioxidants.

peppermint white hot chocolate

No heavy cream is required for this low-calorie version of the classic winter beverage. The bold peppermint extract brilliantly masks the tofu, which packs tons of protein into one single serving! **makes 1 serving**

½ cup silken tofu (I like Mori-Nu)

1 cup milk of choice

1 tablespoon melted cacao butter (if unavailable, this can be omitted for a plain peppermint beverage)

1½ teaspoons xylitol, pure maple syrup, or granulated sugar of choice

pinch pure stevia extract, or additional 1 tablespoon sweetener of choice

½ teaspoon pure vanilla extract

8 drops pure peppermint extract, or more if desired

⅛ teaspoon salt

Blend all ingredients together in a blender, Magic Bullet, or Vitamix until completely smooth. Gently heat on the stove or in the microwave, or drink it cold.

per serving

Calories	160	Fat	13 grams
Fiber	1 gram	Carbs	20 grams
Protein	9 grams	Weight Watchers PointsPlus Value	3

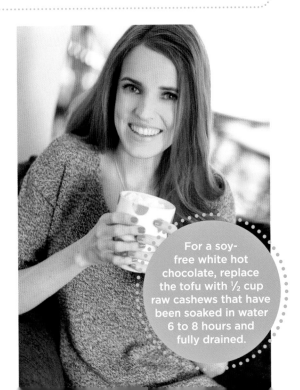

For a soy-free white hot chocolate, replace the tofu with ½ cup raw cashews that have been soaked in water 6 to 8 hours and fully drained.

homemade dairy-free milk

This milk is definitely not just for those who can't drink dairy! Many people simply like to swap this ultra-creamy beverage for cow's milk every now and then as a fun way to shake up their routine. Simple and refreshing, the milk is completely free of preservatives, lactose, and cholesterol. Try making it with any of the following: cashews, macadamia nuts, hazelnuts, pine nuts, Brazil nuts, pistachios, pumpkin seeds, or sunflower seeds. **makes 2 to 3½ cups**

1 cup raw nuts or seeds of choice

2 cups water, plus more for soaking

pinch salt

sweetener of choice, to taste

In a medium bowl, completely cover the nuts or seeds with water. Let soak at room temperature for at least 1 day or up to 2 days. Drain and rinse thoroughly.

In a food processor, blender, or Vitamix, combine the soaked nuts or seeds with 2 cups water and blend until very smooth, scraping down the sides as needed. Line a fine mesh strainer with cheesecloth and set the strainer over a medium container. Strain the milk through the strainer, then fold the cloth over the top. Squeeze out as much liquid as possible. Discard the remaining nutmeat.

Add a pinch of salt to the milk and sweeten to taste. Add more water if a thinner consistency is desired. Store in a covered container in the refrigerator for up to 4 days.

per ½-cup serving

Calories	75	Fat	6.5 grams
Fiber	2 grams	Carbs	2.5 grams
Protein	3 grams	Weight Watchers PointsPlus Value	2

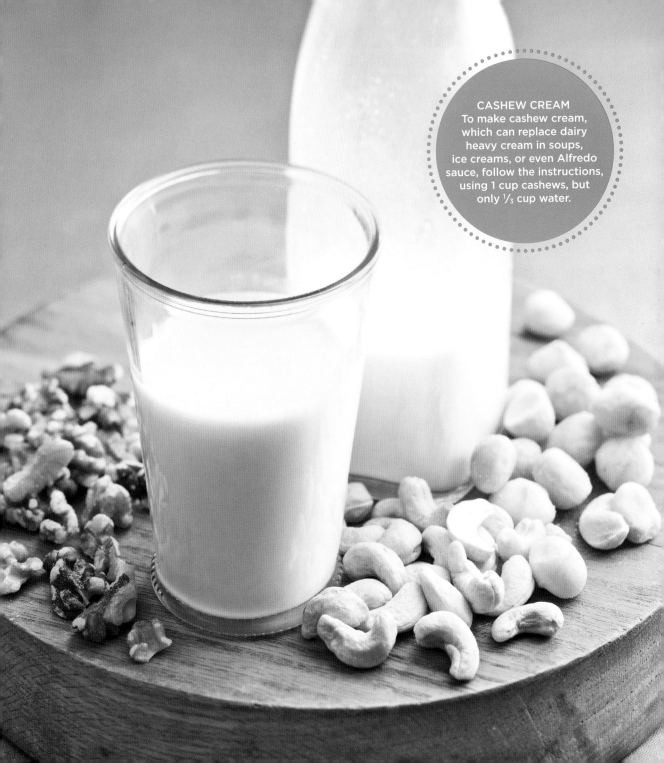

CASHEW CREAM
To make cashew cream, which can replace dairy heavy cream in soups, ice creams, or even Alfredo sauce, follow the instructions, using 1 cup cashews, but only $\frac{1}{3}$ cup water.

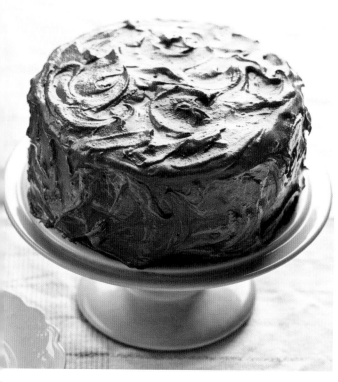
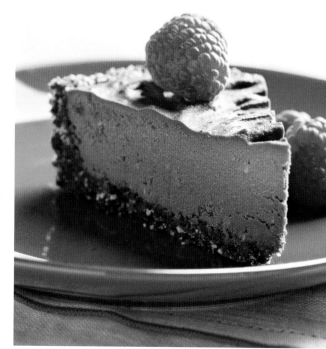
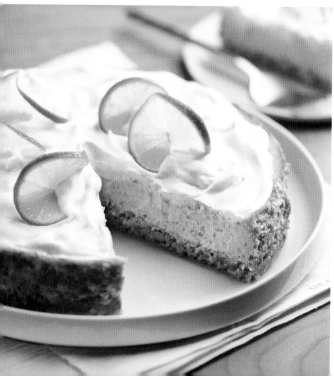
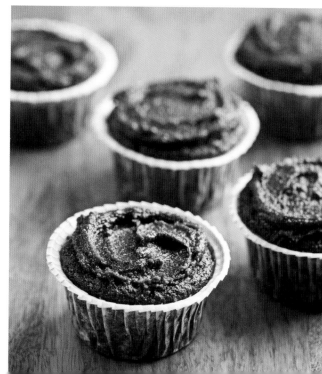

5

pies,
cakes &
cupcakes

deep dish cookie pie

So famous it's been featured on ABC's *Five O'Clock News,* this gooey cookie pie sparked a complete beans-in-dessert revolution on the Internet, inspiring bloggers everywhere to come up with their own cookie, cupcake, and pie recipes using beans instead of flour. With over 1,600 comments on the original post on chocolatecoveredkatie. com, more and more people fall in love with this recipe each day. Will you be next? makes one 10-inch pie (12 servings)

---

2 (15-ounce) cans white beans or garbanzo beans, drained and rinsed well

1½ cups xylitol or granulated sugar of choice

1 cup quick-cooking oats

¼ cup applesauce

3 tablespoons vegetable oil or melted coconut oil

2 teaspoons pure vanilla extract

2 teaspoons baking powder

½ teaspoon baking soda

½ teaspoon salt

1 cup chocolate chips

Preheat the oven to 350 degrees F. Grease a 10-inch springform pan and set aside.

In a high-quality food processor (a blender is not recommended here, but see Note), process all ingredients except chocolate chips until completely smooth. Turn off the food processor and stir in the chocolate chips.

Transfer the batter to the prepared pan. Bake for 35 to 40 minutes, until firm. Remove from the oven and allow to cool for 20 minutes before removing the sides from the pan. Cut into slices, and top with Pure Bliss Vanilla Ice Cream (page 106) if desired.

Refrigerate leftovers in a covered container for up to 4 days. Or freeze for up to a month.

Note: If you must use a blender for this recipe, do so in two batches, which gives all ingredients a chance to evenly blend. This is the only way to achieve the correct texture.

per serving

Calories	200		Fat	8.5 grams
Fiber	4.5 grams		Carbs	27 grams
Protein	5 grams	Weight Watchers PointsPlus Value		5

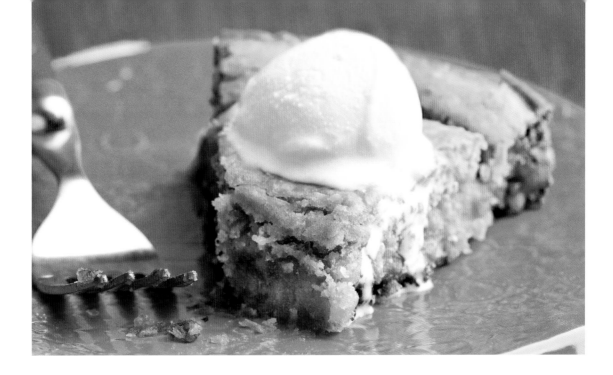

sugar-free deep dish cookie pie

2 (15-ounce) cans white beans or garbanzo beans, drained and rinsed very well

2 cups pitted dates

1 cup quick-cooking oats

²/₃ cup milk of choice

¼ cup applesauce

3 tablespoons coconut or vegetable oil

1 tablespoon pure vanilla extract

2 teaspoons baking powder

½ teaspoon baking soda

¾ teaspoon salt

⅛ teaspoon pure stevia extract

1 cup chocolate chips (for a completely sugar-free pie, be sure to use sugar-free chocolate chips)

Preheat the oven to 350 degrees F. Grease a 10-inch springform pan and set aside.

In a large mixing bowl, stir together all ingredients except chocolate chips.

Transfer about one-third of the mixture to a high-quality food processor (a blender is not recommended here) and blend until completely smooth. Scoop the batter into the prepared pan. Repeat twice, until all of the ingredients have been blended. Stir in the chocolate chips.

Bake for 40 minutes, until firm. Remove from the oven and allow to cool for 20 minutes before removing the sides of the pan. Refrigerate leftovers in a covered container for up to 4 days, or freeze for up to a month.

per serving

Calories	130	Fat	5 grams
Fiber	4 grams	Carbs	23 grams
Protein	2 grams	Weight Watchers PointsPlus Value	4

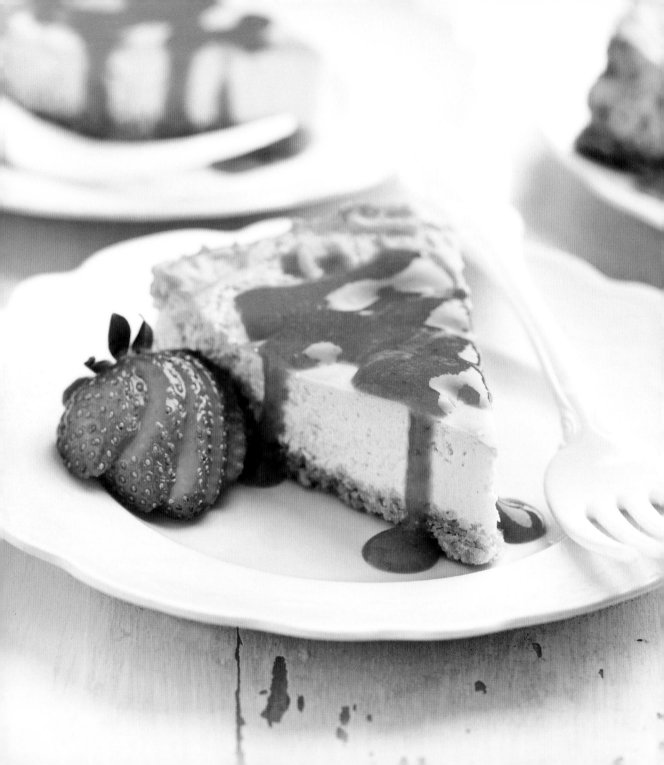

new york–style cheesecake

I'll admit to being somewhat of a cheesecake snob, refusing to eat anything but the smoothest, richest, and most luxurious cheesecake, which absolutely melts in your mouth with every bite. This cheesecake recipe totally fits that bill...You'll never in a million years believe it could possibly be so healthy! makes one 8½-inch cheesecake (10 servings)

2 cups cream cheese (I like Tofutti's non-hydrogenated Better Than Cream Cheese)

6 ounces firm silken tofu (½ of a 12.3-ounce package) (I recommend Mori-Nu)

¼ cup pure maple syrup or raw agave

pinch pure stevia extract, or additional 1 tablespoon sweetener of choice

¼ cup milk of choice

1 tablespoon lemon juice

2 teaspoons pure vanilla extract

¼ teaspoon salt

Oatmeal Cookie Pie Crust (page 197), or prepared 8½-inch pie crust

Preheat the oven to 350 degrees F.

In a food processor, blender, or Vitamix, combine all ingredients and blend until smooth. Be sure not to overblend, as this introduces air into the cheesecake and can cause cracking when baked.

Transfer the filling to the prepared pie crust and bake for 1 hour. Turn off the heat, but do not open the oven door. Allow the cheesecake to continue cooking in the cooling oven for an additional 1 hour. At this point, the cheesecake will still look soft. Refrigerate for at least 8 hours to firm up before slicing.

Just before serving, top with fresh berries if desired, or blend fresh berries with a little sweetener of choice and spoon the mixture over the top of each slice of cheesecake. Cover and refrigerate leftovers for up to 3 days.

per serving

Calories	120		Fat	8 grams
Fiber	0 grams		Carbs	9 grams
Protein	3 grams	Weight Watchers PointsPlus Value	3	

chocolate obsession cake

Moist, rich, and extra chocolaty, this luxurious cake is secretly *packed* with whole grains, probiotics, and antioxidants. Does it look healthy? Trust me, it definitely doesn't taste healthy either!

makes one 8-inch cake (10 servings)

- 1 cup spelt flour, whole wheat pastry flour, or all-purpose flour*
- ³⁄₄ cup xylitol or granulated sugar of choice
- ¹⁄₄ cup plus 2 tablespoons cacao powder or unsweetened cocoa powder
- ¹⁄₂ teaspoon baking soda
- ¹⁄₂ teaspoon salt
- ¹⁄₂ cup mini chocolate chips, optional
- ¹⁄₂ cup carrot juice or milk of choice
- ¹⁄₃ cup plain yogurt of choice (I like WholeSoy or So Delicious cultured coconut milk)
- ¹⁄₄ cup water
- 3 tablespoons vegetable oil or melted coconut oil
- 2 teaspoons pure vanilla extract
- 4-Ingredient Chocolate Frosting (page 191), optional

Preheat the oven to 350 degrees F. Grease an 8-inch round or square baking pan and set aside.

In a large mixing bowl, combine the flour, sugar of choice, cacao powder, baking soda, salt, and chocolate chips (if using) and stir very well.

In a separate mixing bowl, whisk together all remaining ingredients, except frosting. Pour wet ingredients into dry and stir until just evenly combined.

Transfer the batter to the prepared pan. Bake for 25 minutes, until the cake has domed and a toothpick inserted into the center comes out clean. Remove from the oven and allow to cool for at least 10 minutes before removing from the pan.

Frost with 4-Ingredient Chocolate Frosting (page 191) or frosting of choice. If using the 4-Ingredient Chocolate Frosting, this cake is best frosted the day it is served, due to the lack of chemicals and preservatives in the natural frosting. Refrigerate leftovers in a covered container for up to 3 days.

per serving, without frosting

Calories	100		Fat	4 grams
Fiber	3 grams		Carbs	14 grams
Protein	3 grams		Weight Watchers PointsPlus Value	3

*For a gluten-free cake, substitute Bob's Red Mill gluten-free all-purpose baking flour for the flour, and add ¹⁄₂ teaspoon xanthan gum with the flour.

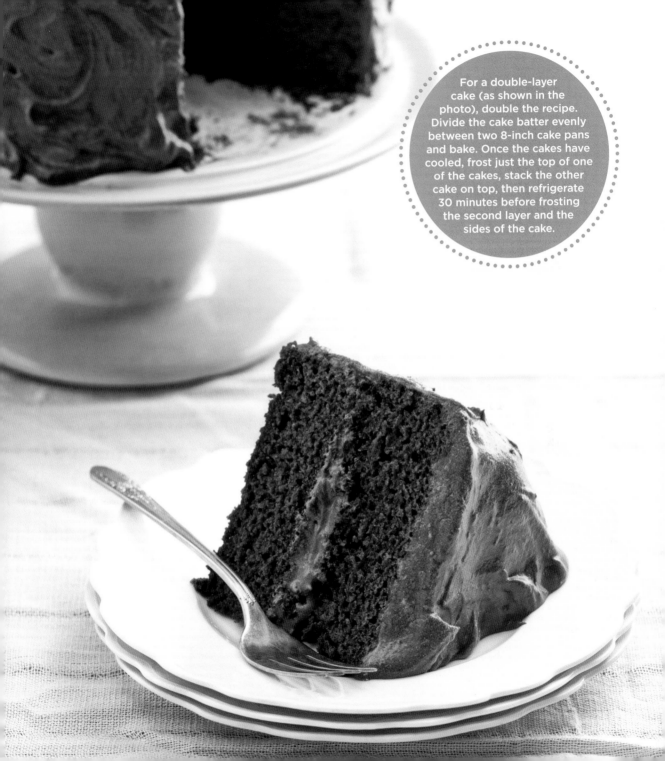

For a double-layer cake (as shown in the photo), double the recipe. Divide the cake batter evenly between two 8-inch cake pans and bake. Once the cakes have cooled, frost just the top of one of the cakes, stack the other cake on top, then refrigerate 30 minutes before frosting the second layer and the sides of the cake.

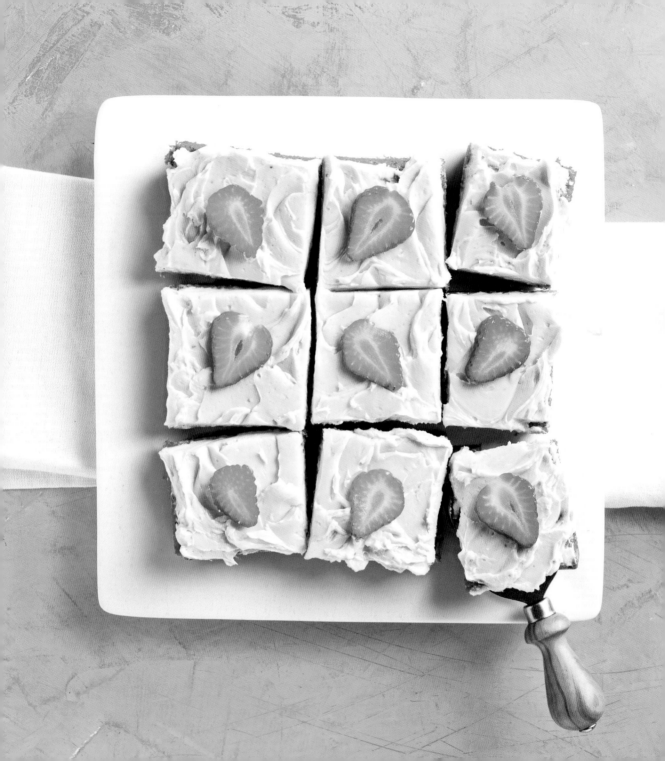

pink princess cake

My younger sister is the world's most devoted fan of the color pink. Visiting her bedroom is like stepping into a Barbie dream house—everything, from the bedspread to the curtains to the walls, is completely saturated in pink. And each year for her birthday, she requests the same thing: a strawberry cake with hot pink frosting. This recipe is dedicated to my sister and to all the pink princesses in the world. makes one 8-inch cake (9 servings)

1½ cups sliced strawberries

3 tablespoons vegetable oil or melted coconut oil

1 tablespoon apple cider vinegar

1½ teaspoons pure vanilla extract

1 cup spelt flour *

½ cup xylitol or granulated sugar of choice

1 teaspoon baking soda

½ teaspoon baking powder

½ teaspoon salt

Strawberry Cupcake Frosting (page 193), optional

Preheat the oven to 350 degrees F. Grease an 8-inch square baking pan and set aside.

In a blender or food processor, blend the strawberries, oil, vinegar, and vanilla until smooth.

In a large mixing bowl, combine all remaining ingredients except the frosting and stir very well. Pour the wet ingredients into the dry and stir until just combined.

Pour the batter into the prepared pan. Bake for 50 minutes, until the cake has risen and a toothpick inserted into the center comes out clean.

If desired, frost with Strawberry Cupcake Frosting (page 193) or frosting of choice just before serving. Refrigerate leftovers in a covered container for up to 3 days.

per serving

Calories	70		Fat	.5 gram
Fiber	5 grams		Carbs	14 grams
Protein	3 grams	Weight Watchers PointsPlus Value		2

*For a gluten-free cake, substitute Bob's Red Mill gluten-free all-purpose baking flour for the flour, and add ½ teaspoon xanthan gum with the flour.

chocolate infinity pie

This chocolate pie might just be my favorite of all the recipes in this entire cookbook, and I could happily eat it every day for breakfast, lunch, and dinner, from now until infinity. **makes one 8½-inch pie (8 servings)**

1 (12.3-ounce) package firm silken tofu (I recommend Mori-Nu)

1⅓ cups chocolate chips, melted (see page 198)

3 tablespoons pure maple syrup or raw agave

2 tablespoons milk of choice

2 teaspoons cacao powder or unsweetened cocoa powder

1 teaspoon pure vanilla extract

scant ⅛ teaspoon salt

Chocolate Cookie Pie Crust (page 194), or prepared 8½-inch pie crust, optional

Process all ingredients except crust in a food processor, blender, or Vitamix until completely smooth. If making with a crust, pour filling into the prepared pie crust. Otherwise, divide the batter among 8 (½-cup) ramekins. Refrigerate uncovered for at least 6 hours to firm up.

Refrigerate leftovers in a covered container for up to 4 days.

per serving

Calories	140	Fat	6 grams
Fiber	4 grams	Carbs	18 grams
Protein	3 grams	Weight Watchers PointsPlus Value	3

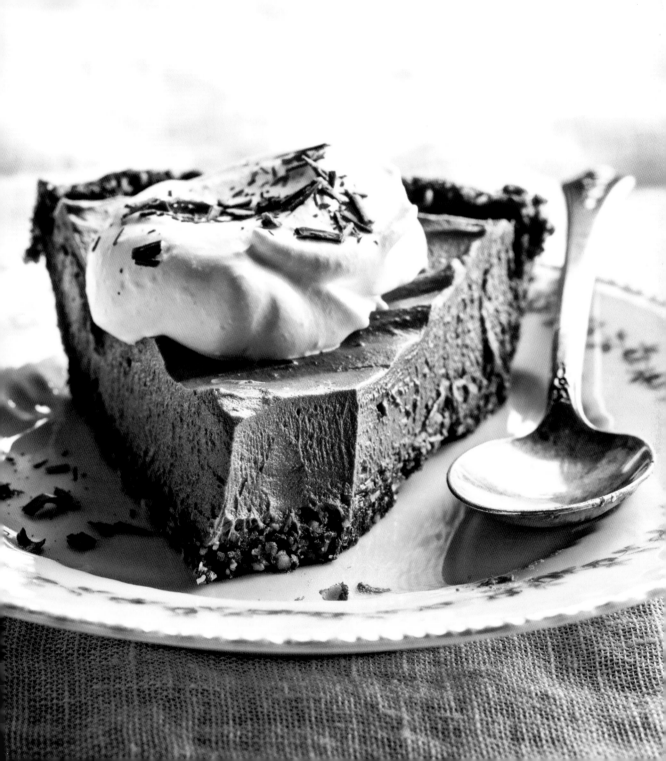

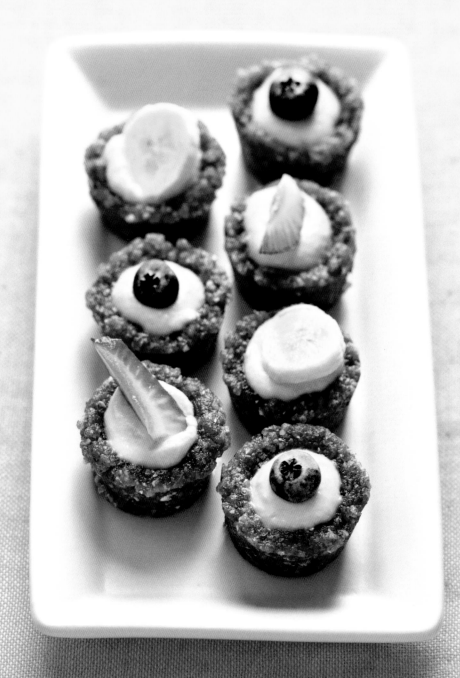

cashew cream mini tarts

Bring these tarts to a dinner party or a fancy afternoon tea. You can make lemon cream tarts by simply replacing 3 tablespoons of the water in the filling with an equal amount of lemon juice.

makes 24 to 26 mini tarts

TART SHELLS
2 cups raw walnuts

1⅓ cups packed pitted dates

½ cup quick-cooking oats

½ teaspoon salt

2 tablespoons water, if needed

FILLING
1 cup raw cashews, soaked in water at room temperature for 6 to 8 hours, then drained and patted dry

½ cup water

½ teaspoon pure vanilla extract

pinch pure stevia extract, or 2 tablespoons sweetener of choice

scant ⅛ teaspoon salt

For the shells: Combine the walnuts, dates, oats, and salt in a high-quality food processor, and process until small crumbles form and the dough begins to stick together in one big ball. If mixture is too dry, add up to 2 tablespoons water and continue to process.

Break off pieces of dough with your hands and press inside one 24-cup or two 12-cup mini muffin tins, pressing down in the middle so that a cup shape is formed. Freeze for 20 minutes, until hardened.

Meanwhile, for the filling: In a high-quality food processor or Vitamix, process the drained cashews with the water, vanilla, stevia, and salt until completely smooth, scraping down the sides occasionally.

Pop the frozen tart shells out of the tin and fill with the cream. Refrigerate until ready to serve. Refrigerate leftovers in a covered container for up to 3 days.

per mini tart (based on 26 tarts)

Calories	110		Fat	7 grams
Fiber	2 grams		Carbs	10 grams
Protein	3.5 grams	Weight Watchers PointsPlus Value		3

cherry peach crumble tart

Ripe peaches, sweet cherries, and a buttery oatmeal crumble combine for one dazzlingly delightful dessert. (Say that three times fast.) The recipe is deceptively simple to make, and it always gets rave reviews.

makes one 8½-inch tart (10 servings)

CRUST

1⅓ cups spelt flour or all-purpose flour*

3 tablespoons xylitol or granulated sugar of choice

pinch pure stevia extract, or additional 1 tablespoon granulated sugar of choice

¼ teaspoon cinnamon

¼ teaspoon salt

¼ cup plus 1 tablespoon vegetable oil or melted coconut oil

1 tablespoon water

FILLING

2 cups peeled and sliced peaches (fresh or thawed frozen)

2 cups cherries (pitted fresh or thawed frozen)

1 tablespoon pure maple syrup or raw agave

CRUMBLES

¼ cup spelt flour or all-purpose flour

¼ cup rolled oats

3 tablespoons brown sugar or coconut sugar

pinch pure stevia extract, or additional 1 tablespoon brown sugar

2 tablespoons melted coconut oil or vegetable oil

⅛ teaspoon salt

For the crust: Preheat the oven to 350 degrees F. Line an 8½-inch springform pan or removable-bottomed tart pan with parchment paper and set aside.

In a large mixing bowl, combine the flour, sugar of choice, stevia, cinnamon, and salt and stir very well. Stir in the oil and water to make a dough. Transfer to the prepared pan and press down. Bake for 12 minutes.

Meanwhile, for the filling: Toss the fruits and maple syrup in a medium mixing bowl and set aside.

For the crumbles: In a small bowl, combine all crumble ingredients and stir until small crumbles form.

Remove the springform pan from the oven and immediately top with the fruit mixture, then evenly sprinkle the crumbles on top. Return the tart to the oven and bake for 35 to 40 minutes, until lightly golden.

Remove from the oven and allow to cool on a wire rack for 20 minutes before removing the pan bottom. Serve with Pure Bliss Vanilla Ice Cream (page 106) if desired.

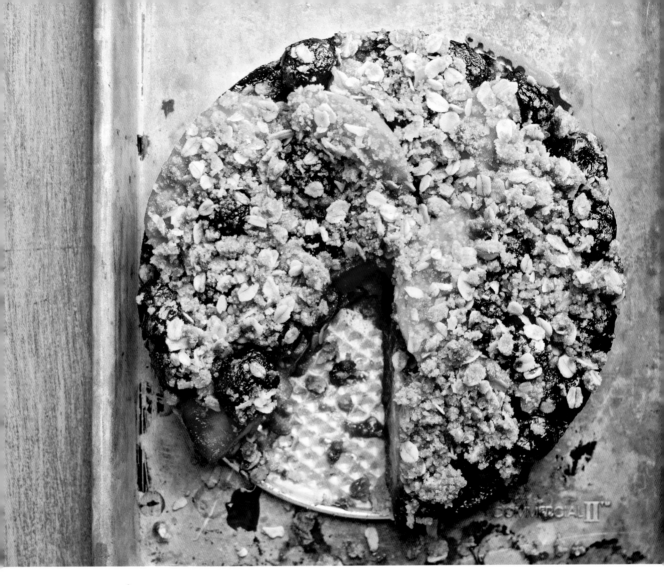

per serving

Calories	225	Fat	10 grams
Fiber	4 grams	Carbs	32.5 grams
Protein	3.5 grams	Weight Watchers PointsPlus Value	4

* For a gluten-free crumble, substitute Bob's Red Mill gluten-free all-purpose baking flour for the flour, and add ¼ teaspoon xanthan gum with the flour.

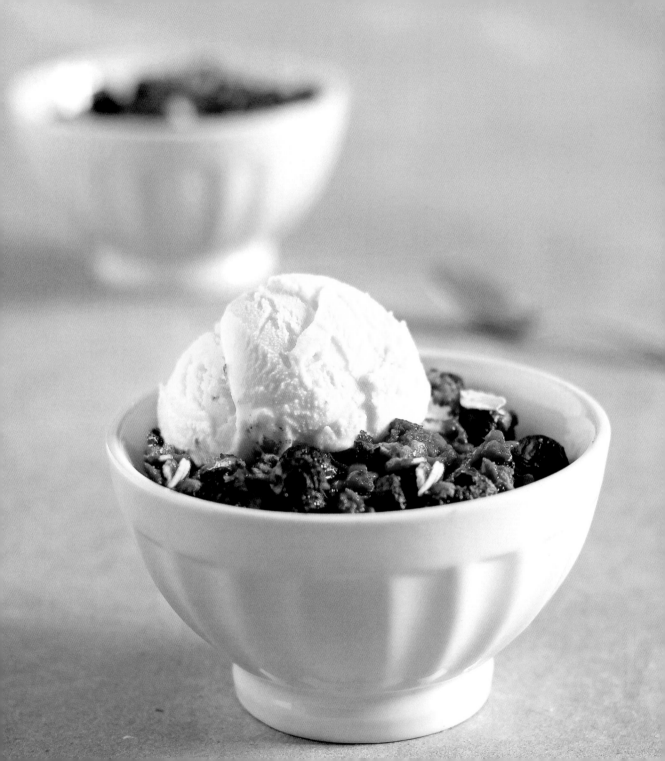

berry oatmeal crumble

Most traditional crumble recipes are heavy on the butter and flour. This lighter and healthier version cuts down on the fat, allowing the fresh raspberries and blueberries to take the spotlight. Feel free to substitute your favorite seasonal fruits—such as diced peaches or pears—for the berries. makes 4 to 6 servings

- 1/2 cup rolled oats
- 1/4 cup plus 1 tablespoon flour of choice (excluding coconut flour)
- 1 teaspoon cinnamon
- 1/2 teaspoon baking soda
- 1/4 teaspoon salt
- 1/16 heaping teaspoon pure stevia extract, or 3 1/2 tablespoons sweetener of choice
- 1/4 cup vegetable oil, melted coconut oil, or buttery spread (I like Earth Balance), optional
- 2 cups raspberries (fresh or thawed frozen)
- 2 cups blueberries (fresh or thawed frozen)
- 1 1/2 teaspoons lemon juice
- 1 teaspoon pure vanilla extract

Preheat the oven to 350 degrees F. Grease an 8-inch square baking pan and set aside.

In a large mixing bowl, combine the oats, flour, cinnamon, baking soda, salt, and stevia. If a richer crumble is desired, go ahead and add the oil or cut in the buttery spread until crumbles form. In a medium mixing bowl, stir together the berries, lemon juice, and vanilla. Pour the wet ingredients into the dry mixture and stir to combine.

Transfer to the prepared pan and spread evenly. Bake for 25 minutes, until golden.

Serve with Pure Bliss Vanilla Ice Cream (page 106) if desired. Refrigerate leftovers in a covered container for up to 4 days.

per serving

Calories	90	Fat	1 gram
Fiber	6 grams	Carbs	20 grams
Protein	3 grams	Weight Watchers PointsPlus Value	1

red velvet fudge pie

This is a romantic and elegant dessert for that special someone in your life. If you don't have a special someone in your life? Great! More for you! **makes one 8½-inch pie (12 servings)**

2 cups raspberries (fresh or thawed frozen)

½ cup plus 1 tablespoon cacao powder or unsweetened cocoa powder

¾ cup melted coconut butter

5½ tablespoons pure maple syrup or raw agave

⅛ teaspoon plus ¹⁄₁₆ teaspoon salt

Chocolate Cookie Pie Crust (page 194), optional

Combine all ingredients except optional crust in a food processor, blender, or Vitamix and process until completely smooth. If using a crust, spread the crust into the bottom of an 8½-inch springform pan and press down firmly. Using a spatula, spread the filling either on top of the crust or evenly into the pan.

Freeze at least 3 hours, until the filling firms up to a fudge-like texture.

Refrigerate leftovers in a covered container for up to a week or freeze for up to a month. If freezing, thaw the pie for 20 minutes, or until it once again has a fudge-like texture, before slicing and serving.

per serving

Calories	135	Fat	9 grams
Fiber	5.5 grams	Carbs	14 grams
Protein	2 grams	Weight Watchers PointsPlus Value	4

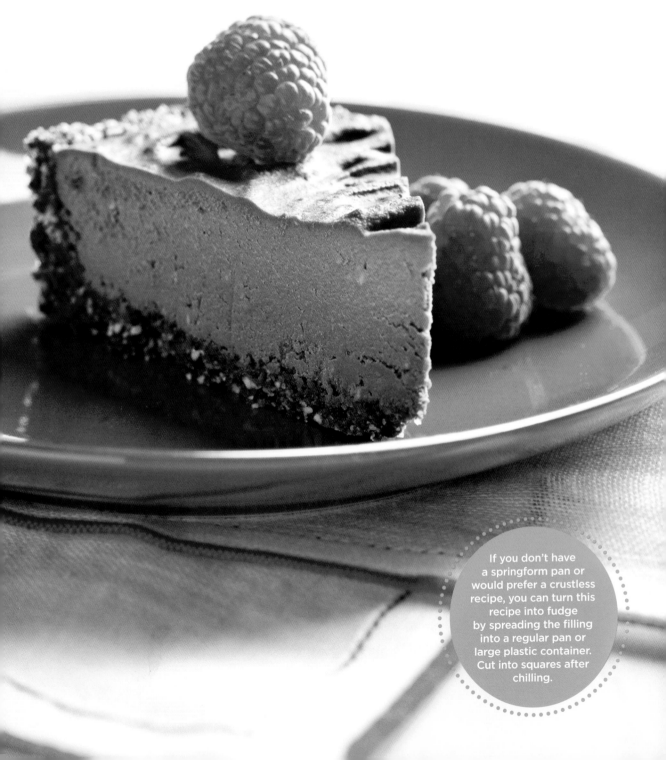

If you don't have
a springform pan or
would prefer a crustless
recipe, you can turn this
recipe into fudge
by spreading the filling
into a regular pan or
large plastic container.
Cut into squares after
chilling.

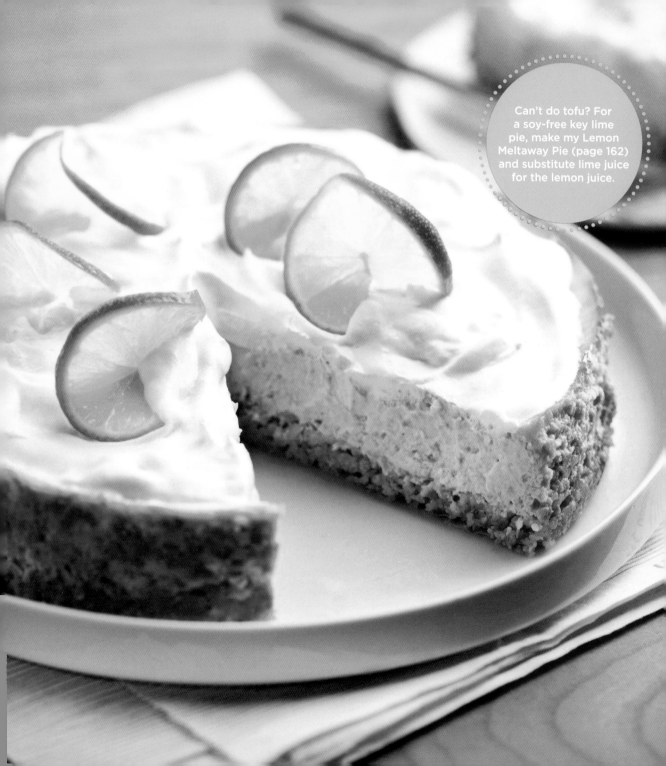

Can't do tofu? For a soy-free key lime pie, make my Lemon Meltaway Pie (page 162) and substitute lime juice for the lemon juice.

key lime pie cheesecake

How are you possibly supposed to choose between New York cheesecake and Florida key lime pie? Oh, but why choose at all? This recipe lets you have both! makes one 8½-inch cheesecake (12 servings)

2 (12.3-ounce) packages firm silken tofu (I recommend Mori-Nu) (see note on opposite page)

½ cup key lime juice or regular lime juice if key lime is not available

¼ cup pure maple syrup

⅛ teaspoon pure stevia extract, or ¼ cup granulated sugar of choice

⅓ cup melted coconut butter

1½ teaspoons pure vanilla extract

½ teaspoon salt

Oatmeal Cookie Pie Crust (page 197), or prepared 8½-inch pie crust

Preheat the oven to 350 degrees F.

Combine all ingredients except crust in a food processor, blender, or Vitamix and blend until just smooth. Be sure not to over-blend the filling, as this introduces air into the cheesecake and can cause cracking when baked.

Transfer the filling to the prepared crust. Bake for 65 minutes, until the top of the cheesecake has set. Remove from the oven and allow to cool completely. It will still look soft, but this is okay. Refrigerate uncovered for at least 8 hours, until the texture has firmed up considerably.

If using the Oatmeal Cookie Pie Crust, gently run a knife around the side of the pan to loosen before taking off the springform. Cut into slices, and serve with Coconut Whipped Cream (page 183) if desired. Cover and refrigerate leftovers for up to 3 days.

per serving

Calories	95	Fat	5.5 grams
Fiber	5 grams	Carbs	7.5 grams
Protein	2 grams	Weight Watchers PointsPlus Value	2

miss scarlet strawberry pie

During the summers when I was growing up, my family spent many evenings on the patio playing board games such as Trivial Pursuit and Clue (I insisted on being Miss Scarlet every single time) and eating whatever "made from scratch" dessert my cooking-enthusiast mother had prepared earlier in the day. We always got especially excited whenever her strawberry pie was on the menu. It's the quintessential dessert for a hot summer's night. makes one 8½-inch pie (8 servings)

Oatmeal Cookie Pie Crust (page 197), or prepared 8½-inch pie crust

1 pound fresh whole strawberries, stems cut off, plus ⅔ cup finely chopped fresh strawberries

2 teaspoons grated lemon zest

¼ cup lemon juice

pinch pure stevia extract, or 1 tablespoon sweetener of choice

⅓ cup pure maple syrup or raw agave

1 envelope vegetarian gelatin (I like Jel Dessert from Natural Desserts, which can be found at Whole Foods or online)

3½ tablespoons cold water

Fill the pie crust with the whole strawberries, cut side down, and set aside.

In a saucepan, stir together the chopped strawberries, lemon zest and juice, and stevia. Cook over medium-low heat for 5 minutes, stirring once or twice. Add the maple syrup, lower the heat, and simmer for 2 minutes.

In a small bowl, mix the gelatin with the cold water until fully dissolved. Immediately pour the mixture into the saucepan, increase the heat to high, and bring to a boil. As soon as the mixture begins to boil, turn the heat off. Let cool for 20 minutes.

Pour the cooled mixture into the pie crust. Refrigerate for at least 5 hours, allowing the pie to set.

Top with Coconut Whipped Cream (page 183) if desired. Cover and refrigerate leftovers for up to 3 days.

per serving

Calories	55	Fat	0 grams
Fiber	6 grams	Carbs	14 grams
Protein	.5 gram	Weight Watchers PointsPlus Value	1

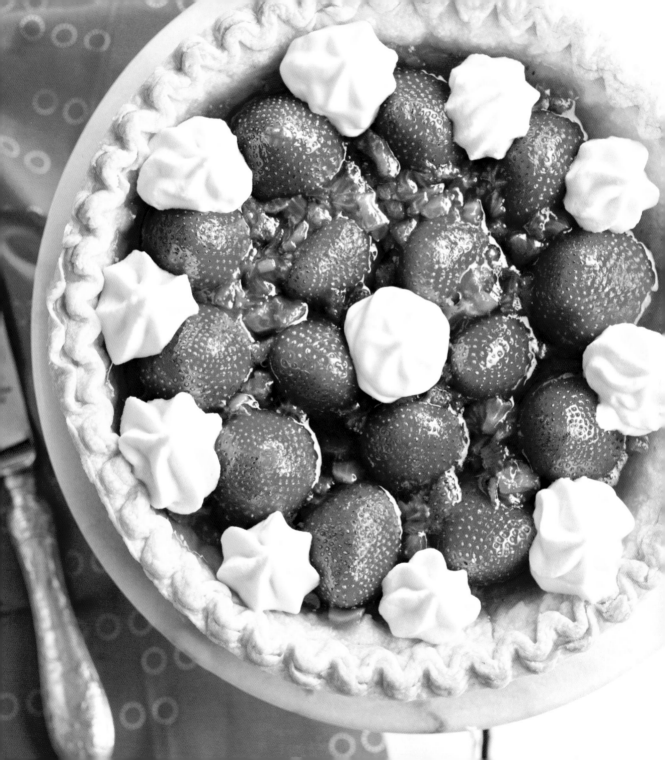

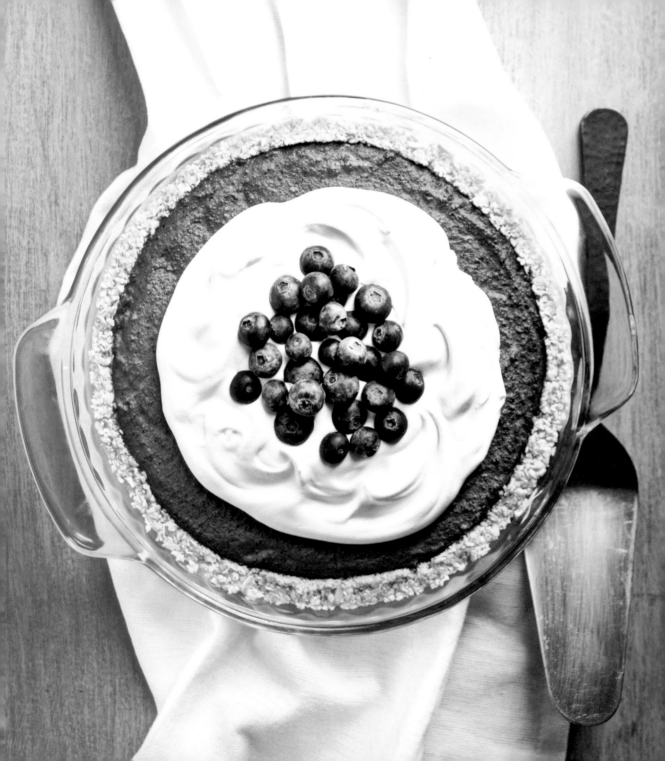

blueberry silk pie

This mousse-like pie is the kind of dessert you'd expect to encounter at a glamorous and exclusive Hollywood banquet. It is sleek, silky, and opulent, like the culinary answer to a sparkling diamond ring.

makes one 8½-inch pie (12 servings)

1½ cups raw macadamia nuts

2 cups blueberries

⅓ cup melted virgin coconut oil

1½ teaspoons pure vanilla extract

⅛ teaspoon pure stevia extract, or ¼ cup sweetener of choice

⅛ teaspoon salt

Oatmeal Cookie Pie Crust (page 197), or prepared pie crust

In a medium bowl, cover the macadamia nuts with water and soak for 6 to 8 hours. Drain completely.

Combine the nuts and all remaining ingredients except the crust in a high-powered food processor or Vitamix. If using stevia, add 3 tablespoons water. Process until the ingredients are completely smooth.

Transfer the filling to the prepared pie crust, smooth the top of the pie, and freeze at least 6 hours, until firm. Top with Coconut Whipped Cream (page 183) and fresh blueberries if desired. Refrigerate leftovers in a covered container for up to 5 days, or freeze for up to a month. If freezing, thaw the pie for 20 minutes, or until it once again has a smooth texture, before slicing and serving.

per serving

Calories	180		Fat	18 grams
Fiber	3 grams		Carbs	5.5 grams
Protein	1.5 grams		Weight Watchers PointsPlus Value	5

lemon meltaway pie

Want to shock your guests at your next dinner party? Watch them devour this pie *before* you reveal the healthy hidden ingredient—cauliflower! Be sure to have a camera on hand to capture their astonished expressions.

makes one 8½-inch pie (10 servings)

1 cup raw cashews or macadamia nuts

2 cups loosely packed frozen cauliflower, thawed completely (see note on opposite page)

$\frac{1}{3}$ cup melted virgin coconut oil

$\frac{1}{4}$ cup plus 2 tablespoons lemon juice

1 tablespoon pure vanilla extract

$\frac{1}{8}$ teaspoon pure stevia extract, or $\frac{1}{4}$ cup pure maple syrup or raw agave

$\frac{1}{8}$ teaspoon plus $\frac{1}{16}$ teaspoon salt

Oatmeal Cookie Pie Crust (page 197), or prepared pie crust

In a medium bowl, cover the nuts with water and soak for 6 to 8 hours. Drain completely.

Combine the nuts and all remaining ingredients except crust in a high-powered food processor or Vitamix. If using stevia, add 3 tablespoons water. Process on high until completely smooth.

Transfer the filling to the prepared pie crust and freeze for at least 3 hours, until firm.

Refrigerate leftovers in a covered container for up to a week or freeze for up to a month. If freezing, thaw the pie for 20 minutes, or until it once again has a smooth texture, before slicing and serving.

per serving

Calories	180		Fat	17 grams
Fiber	2 grams		Carbs	7 grams
Protein	3.5 grams	Weight Watchers PointsPlus Value		5

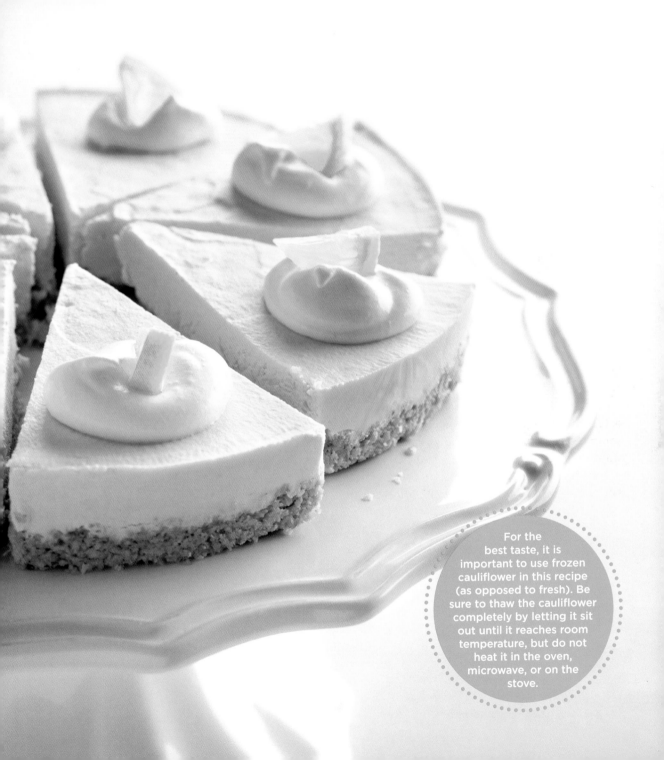

For the best taste, it is important to use frozen cauliflower in this recipe (as opposed to fresh). Be sure to thaw the cauliflower completely by letting it sit out until it reaches room temperature, but do not heat it in the oven, microwave, or on the stove.

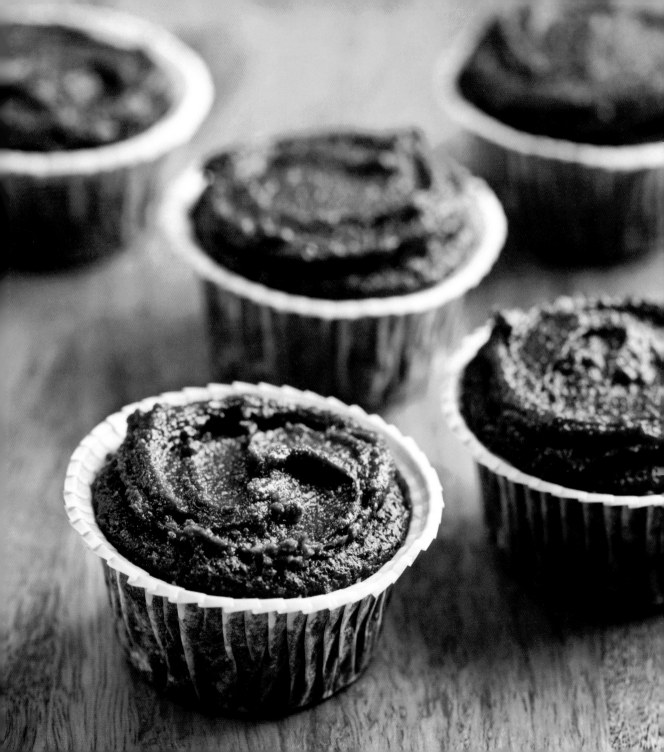

chocolate banana bread cupcakes

The only thing better than homemade banana bread cupcakes right out of the oven is homemade *chocolate* banana bread cupcakes right out of the oven. Everything is better with chocolate. (Yes, everything.)

makes 10 cupcakes

- ½ cup milk of choice
- ½ cup over-ripe mashed banana (measured after mashing)
- 3½ tablespoons vegetable oil or coconut oil
- 2½ teaspoons pure vanilla extract

- 2 teaspoons apple cider vinegar
- ¾ cup spelt flour or all-purpose flour*
- ½ cup xylitol or granulated sugar of choice
- pinch pure stevia extract, or additional 1 tablespoon granulated sugar of choice

- ¼ cup cacao powder or unsweetened cocoa powder
- ½ teaspoon baking soda
- ½ teaspoon baking powder
- ⅜ teaspoon salt
- ½ cup chocolate chips, optional

Preheat the oven to 350 degrees F. Grease 10 cups of a muffin tin, or line with cupcake liners, and set aside. In a medium mixing bowl, whisk together the milk, mashed banana, oil, vanilla, and vinegar. Set aside for at least 5 minutes.

In a large mixing bowl, combine all remaining ingredients and stir very well. Pour wet ingredients into dry and stir until just evenly mixed.

Portion the batter evenly among the muffin cups, being sure to fill each cup only halfway, as the cupcakes will rise considerably as they bake. Bake for 23 to 25 minutes, until cupcakes have risen and domed and a toothpick inserted into a center comes out clean.

Take the cupcakes out of the oven and allow to cool for 10 minutes before removing from the tin. If desired, frost with Healthy Chocolate *Not*ella (page 187) just before serving. Refrigerate unfrosted leftover cupcakes in a covered container for up to 4 days.

per cupcake

Calories	85		Fat	5 grams
Fiber	2 grams		Carbs	10 grams
Protein	2 grams	Weight Watchers PointsPlus Value		2

*For gluten-free cupcakes, substitute Bob's Red Mill gluten-free all-purpose baking flour for the flour, and add ½ teaspoon xantham gum with the flour.

coconut cloud cupcakes

With their out-of-this-world coconut flavor and fluffy texture, these cupcakes are guaranteed to quickly disappear before your very eyes. Add a little rum extract and you've got yourself a piña colada in a cupcake! **makes 10 cupcakes**

- ½ cup milk of choice
- ½ cup crushed pineapple, drained
- 3½ tablespoons vegetable oil or melted coconut oil
- 2 teaspoons apple cider vinegar
- 2½ teaspoons pure vanilla extract
- ½ teaspoon rum extract, optional
- 1 cup spelt flour or all-purpose flour*
- ½ cup xylitol or granulated sugar of choice
- pinch pure stevia extract, or additional 1 tablespoon granulated sugar of choice
- ½ teaspoon baking soda
- ½ teaspoon baking powder
- ⅜ teaspoon salt

Preheat the oven to 350 degrees F. Grease 10 cups of a muffin tin, or line with cupcake liners, and set aside.

In a medium mixing bowl, whisk together the milk, pineapple, oil, vinegar, vanilla, and rum extract (if desired). Allow to sit at room temperature for at least 5 minutes.

In a large mixing bowl, combine remaining ingredients and stir very well. Pour wet ingredients into dry and stir until just evenly mixed.

Portion the batter evenly among the muffin cups, being sure to fill each cup only halfway, as the cupcakes will rise considerably as they bake. Bake for 20 minutes, until cupcakes have risen and domed and a toothpick inserted into a center comes out clean.

Take the cupcakes out of the oven and allow to cool for 10 minutes before removing from the tin.

If you like, frost cupcakes with Coconut Whipped Cream (page 183) and sprinkle with shredded coconut just before serving. Refrigerate unfrosted leftover cupcakes in a covered container for up to 4 days.

per cupcake

Calories	85	Fat	3 grams
Fiber	2 grams	Carbs	13 grams
Protein	2 grams	Weight Watchers PointsPlus Value	2

*For gluten-free cupcakes, substitute Bob's Red Mill gluten-free all-purpose baking flour, and add ½ teaspoon xantham gum with the flour.

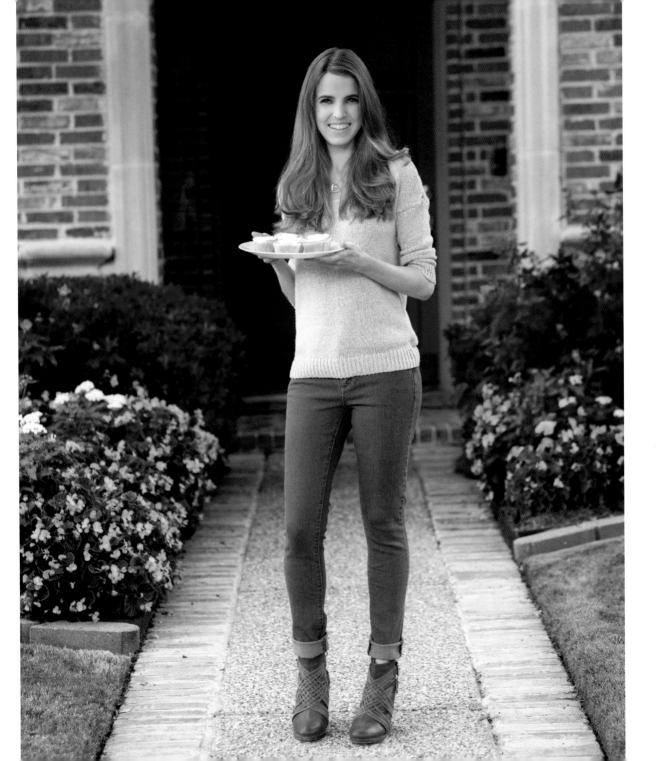

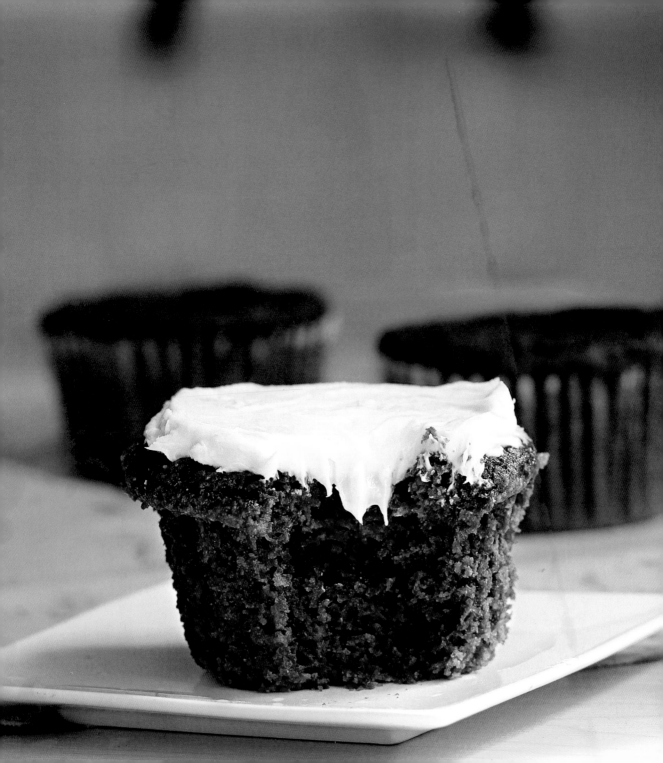

chocolate zucchini cupcakes

The healthy addition of zucchini to these cupcakes makes them incredibly moist. But as soon as you sample the deeply chocolaty finished product, all thoughts of vegetables are immediately forgotten.

makes 10 cupcakes

1¼ cups spelt flour or all-purpose flour*

½ cup xylitol or granulated sugar of choice

pinch pure stevia extract, or additional 2 tablespoons granulated sugar of choice

¼ cup plus 2 tablespoons cacao powder or unsweetened cocoa powder

½ teaspoon baking soda

¾ teaspoon baking powder

⅜ teaspoon salt

1 cup finely grated zucchini

½ cup applesauce

⅓ cup vegetable oil or melted coconut oil

¼ cup plain yogurt of choice (I like WholeSoy or So Delicious cultured coconut milk)

2 teaspoons pure vanilla extract

½ cup mini chocolate chips, optional

Preheat the oven to 350 degrees F. Grease 10 cups of a muffin tin, or line with cupcake liners, and set aside.

In a large mixing bowl, combine the flour, sugar of choice, stevia, cacao powder, baking soda, baking powder, and salt and stir very well.

In a medium mixing bowl, whisk together all remaining ingredients. Pour wet ingredients into dry and stir until just evenly mixed.

Portion the batter evenly among the muffin cups. Bake for 20 minutes, until cupcakes have risen and domed and a toothpick inserted into a center comes out clean.

Take the cupcakes out of the oven and allow to cool for 10 minutes before removing from the tin.

If desired, frost with Healthier Cream Cheese Frosting (page 192) just before serving. Refrigerate unfrosted leftover cupcakes in a covered container for up to 4 days.

per cupcake

Calories	135	Fat	7.5 grams
Fiber	4 grams	Carbs	15 grams
Protein	3.5 grams	Weight Watchers PointsPlus Value	4

*For gluten-free cupcakes, substitute Bob's Red Mill gluten-free all-purpose baking flour, and add ½ teaspoon xantham gum with the flour.

chocolate birthday cake pops

This is one dessert on which parents and children can agree. Kids go crazy for the flavor of these chocolaty pops, while their parents love how healthy they are. **makes 24 to 28 cake pops**

CAKE
1/2 cup spelt flour or all-purpose flour

1/2 cup xylitol or granulated sugar of choice

3 tablespoons cacao powder or unsweetened cocoa powder

1/4 teaspoon baking soda

1/4 teaspoon salt

1/4 cup mini chocolate chips, optional

1/4 cup carrot juice or milk of choice

3 tablespoons plain yogurt of choice (I like WholeSoy or So Delicious cultured coconut milk)

2 tablespoons water

1 1/2 tablespoons vegetable oil or melted coconut oil

1 teaspoon pure vanilla extract

COATING
3 tablespoons cacao powder or unsweetened cocoa powder

2 1/2 tablespoons melted virgin coconut oil

1 1/2 tablespoons pure maple syrup or raw agave

lollipop sticks, found in the baking section of a grocery or craft store

For the cake: Preheat the oven to 350 degrees F. Grease an 8-inch round or square baking pan and set aside.

In a large mixing bowl, combine the flour, sugar of choice, cacao powder, baking soda, salt, and chocolate chips (if using) and stir very well.

In a medium mixing bowl, whisk together all remaining cake ingredients. Pour wet ingredients into dry and stir until just combined.

Transfer the batter to the prepared cake pan. Bake for 15 minutes, until a toothpick inserted into the center of the cake comes out clean. Remove from the oven and allow to cool for at least 20 minutes.

For the coating: Mix all ingredients together in a deep cup or bowl.

Line a large plate with parchment or waxed paper. Using a small cookie scoop or your hands, break off small pieces of cake and roll into tight balls. Place each ball on the prepared plate.

Place a cake ball on a spoon and dip into the coating mixture, swirling to coat. Return to the plate and insert a lollipop stick into the middle.

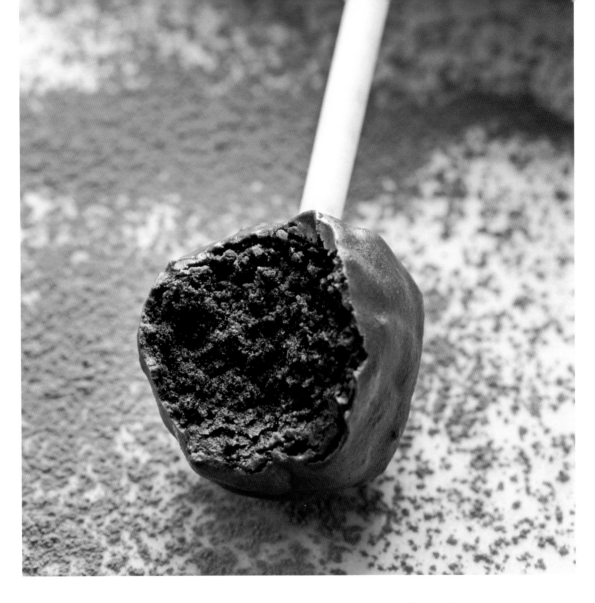

Repeat to coat all the cake balls. Place the plate in the refrigerator for 15 to 20 minutes, until the coating hardens. Cake pops should be stored in the refrigerator in a covered container until ready to serve, and leftovers will last for up to 4 days.

per cake pop with coating

Calories	30	Fat	2 grams
Fiber	1 gram	Carbs	3.5 grams
Protein	.5 gram	Weight Watchers PointsPlus Value	1

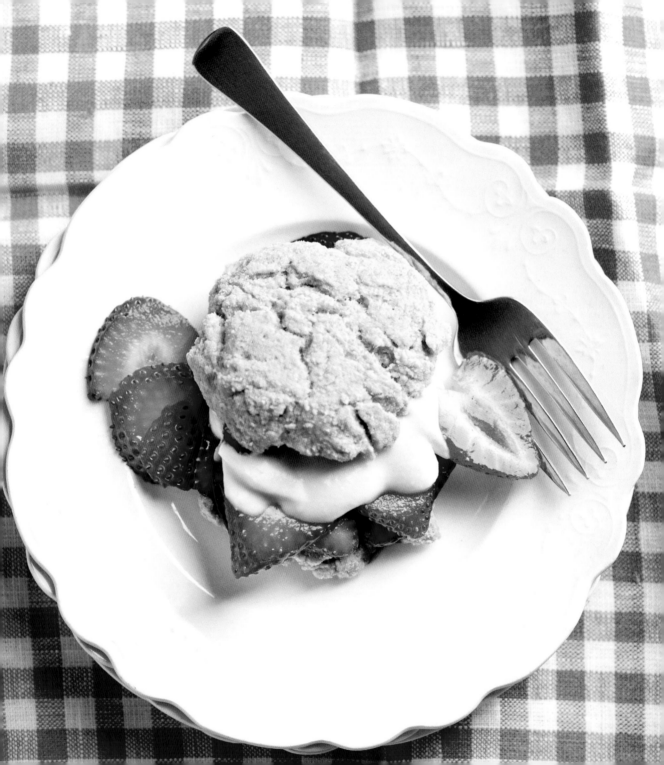

strawberry shortcakes

As a true child of the 1980s, I owned more than my fair share of Strawberry Shortcake dolls. (Not to mention Care Bears, Cabbage Patch Kids, and My Little Ponies…) When I found out there was an actual dessert called "strawberry shortcake," I was overjoyed and immediately set up an elaborate tea party for my dolls. Then I spent the afternoon feeding them—and myself!—strawberry shortcake piled high with whipped cream, in true Katie fashion.

makes 10 shortcakes

2 cups spelt flour or all-purpose flour*

2 tablespoons xylitol or granulated sugar of choice

1 tablespoon baking powder

1 teaspoon salt

1 cup full-fat canned coconut milk or Cashew Cream (page 135)

2 tablespoons vegetable oil or melted coconut oil

2 teaspoons pure vanilla extract

all-fruit jam, for serving

sliced strawberries, for serving

Coconut Whipped Cream (page 183), for serving

Preheat the oven to 350 degrees F. Grease a baking sheet and set aside.

In a large mixing bowl, combine the flour, sugar of choice, baking powder, and salt and stir very well.

In a small mixing bowl, stir together the milk, oil, and vanilla. Pour wet ingredients into dry and mix until just combined.

Drop 10 mounds of dough (3 to 4 tablespoons each) onto the prepared baking sheet, at least 2 inches apart. Bake for 12 minutes, until golden brown. Remove from the oven and allow to cool for 5 minutes.

Slice the shortcakes in half and spread a layer of jam on the bottom halves. Top with the strawberries and whipped cream. Add the shortcake tops.

per shortcake

Calories	160		Fat	8 grams
Fiber	4 grams		Carbs	19 grams
Protein	4 grams	Weight Watchers PointsPlus Value	4	

*For gluten-free shortcakes, substitute Bob's Red Mill gluten-free all-purpose baking flour for the flour, and add ½ teaspoon xantham gum with the flour.

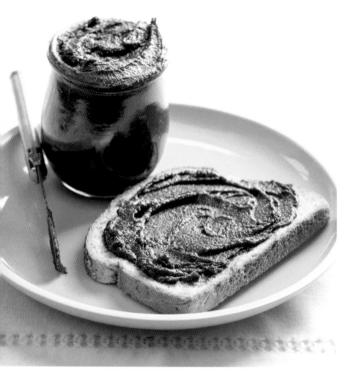
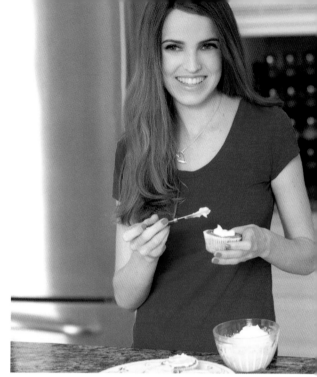
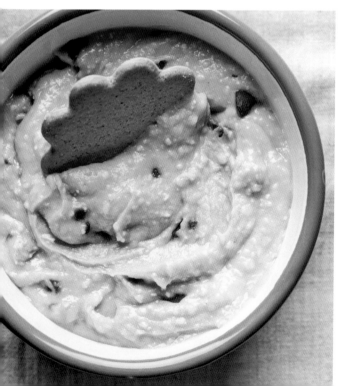
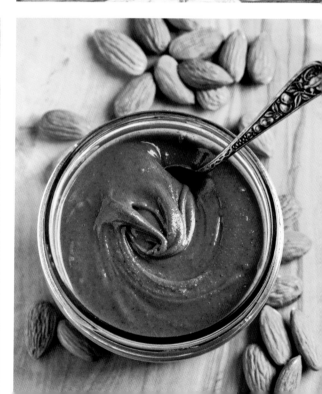

6 puddings, dips, frostings & more

peanut butter fudge brownie dip

Serve this decadent party dip with pretzels, banana slices, fresh strawberries, apples, or graham crackers; spread it on toast or pancakes; or simply eat it with a spoon! makes about 2½ cups

1 (15-ounce) can black beans, drained and rinsed well

½ cup peanut butter or allergy-friendly alternative

3½ tablespoons cacao powder or unsweetened cocoa powder

⅓ cup pure maple syrup or raw agave

1/16 teaspoon pure stevia extract, or 2 tablespoons additional sweetener of choice

2 teaspoons pure vanilla extract

¼ teaspoon salt

up to 3 tablespoons milk of choice

chocolate chips or homemade chocolate chips (see page 198), optional

In a high-quality food processor (a blender is not recommended here, but see Note), blend the black beans, peanut butter, cacao powder, maple syrup, stevia, vanilla, and salt until the texture is completely smooth. Add milk, if needed, for smoother blending. Transfer to a medium bowl. Stir in chocolate chips if desired.

Refrigerate leftovers in a covered container for up to 4 days.

Note: **If you must use a blender for this recipe, do so in two batches, which gives all the ingredients a chance to evenly blend. This is the only way to achieve the correct texture.**

per 1 tablespoon

Calories	30	Fat	1.5 grams
Fiber	1 gram	Carbs	3.5 grams
Protein	1.5 grams	Weight Watchers PointsPlus Value	1

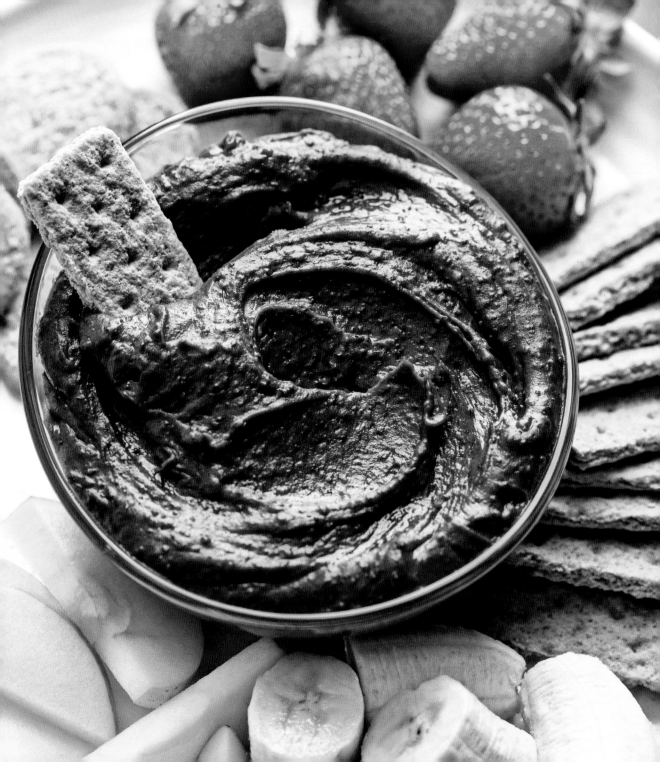

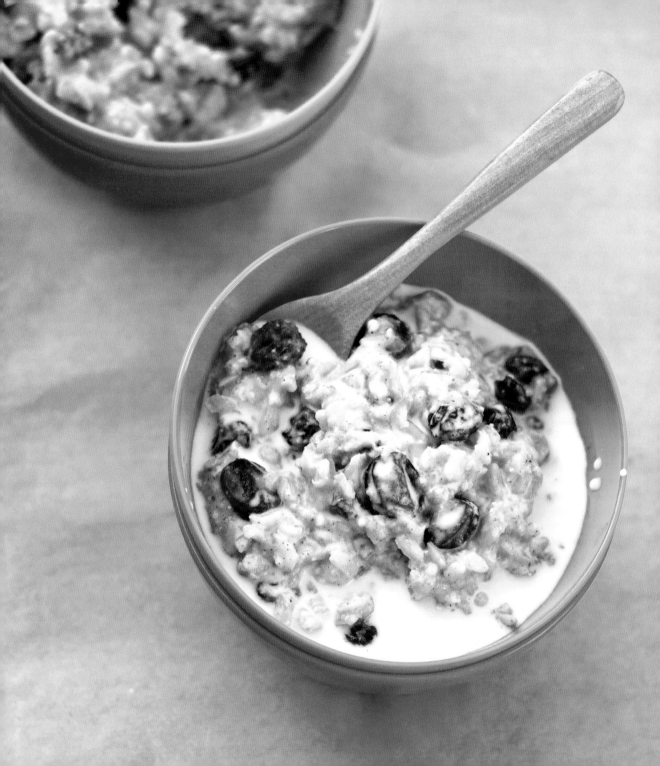

classic rice pudding

Nothing says "comfort food" quite like a simple bowl of creamy rice pudding. While traditional rice pudding is often alarmingly high in calories, fat, and cholesterol, there's thankfully a trick that allows you to cut out a *significant* number of calories without sacrificing any of the taste or texture: Use twice the amount of milk, and cook the rice twice so it thickens more and more as it soaks up all the liquid. The result is a remarkably thick and creamy rice pudding that doesn't have any heavy cream whatsoever! makes 4 to 6 servings

1 cup uncooked brown or white rice

2½ cups plus ⅔ cup (or more as needed) milk of choice, divided

½ teaspoon salt

½ cup raisins, optional

2 teaspoons pure vanilla extract

1 teaspoon cinnamon

¼ teaspoon pure stevia extract, or ½ cup sweetener of choice (or more if omitting raisins)

Combine the rice, 2½ cups milk of choice, and salt in a medium saucepan. Bring to a boil over high heat. As soon as the mixture begins to boil, add the raisins if using, cover the pot, and lower the heat. Simmer until the mixture thickens to a pudding consistency. This can take anywhere from 10 minutes to 50 minutes, depending on the variety of rice you used. (Brown rice takes longer than white, and long-grain takes longer than Arborio.)

Add the ⅔ cup milk of choice and return to a boil. Turn off the heat, but leave the saucepan completely covered and let sit until the milk is absorbed and the rice becomes thick, fluffy, and creamy, about 20 minutes. If the rice looks dry as opposed to creamy after this amount of

time (which will also depend on the variety of rice used), add more milk of choice and stir until the pudding becomes creamy.

Add the vanilla, cinnamon, and stevia. Serve either cold or hot, for a snack or even for breakfast. Refrigerate leftovers in a covered container for up to 4 days. Stir in additional milk before serving to make up for the evaporation that occurs as the pudding sits in the fridge.

per serving

Calories	130	Fat	2 grams
Fiber	2 grams	Carbs	20 grams
Protein	3 grams	Weight Watchers PointsPlus Value	3

chocolate chia power pudding

Chia seeds might just be the ultimate superfood. They contain fiber, calcium, and omega-3s, and have the ability to lower blood pressure, keep you hydrated, and even reduce food cravings. With this chocolate pudding, there's never been a more delicious way to eat your way to good health! **makes 3 to 4 servings**

2¼ cups milk of choice

⅔ cup chia seeds

¼ cup cacao powder or unsweetened cocoa powder

1 teaspoon pure vanilla extract

sweetener of choice, to taste

¼ teaspoon salt

handful chocolate chips or homemade chocolate chips (see page 198), optional

Stir all ingredients except chocolate chips together in a medium bowl. Refrigerate overnight, to thicken. Stir in chocolate chips, if using, just before serving.

per serving

Calories	100		Fat	8 grams
Fiber	9 grams		Carbs	11 grams
Protein	6 grams	Weight Watchers PointsPlus Value	3

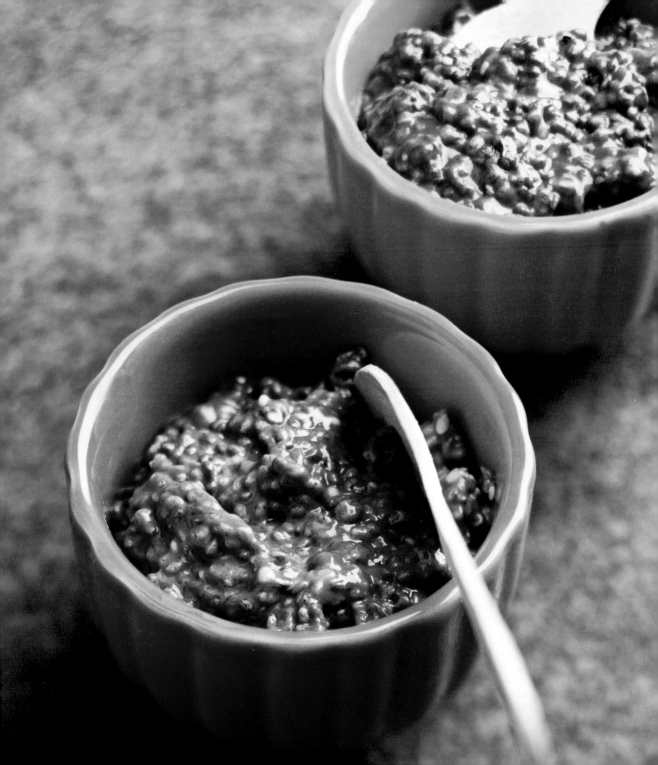

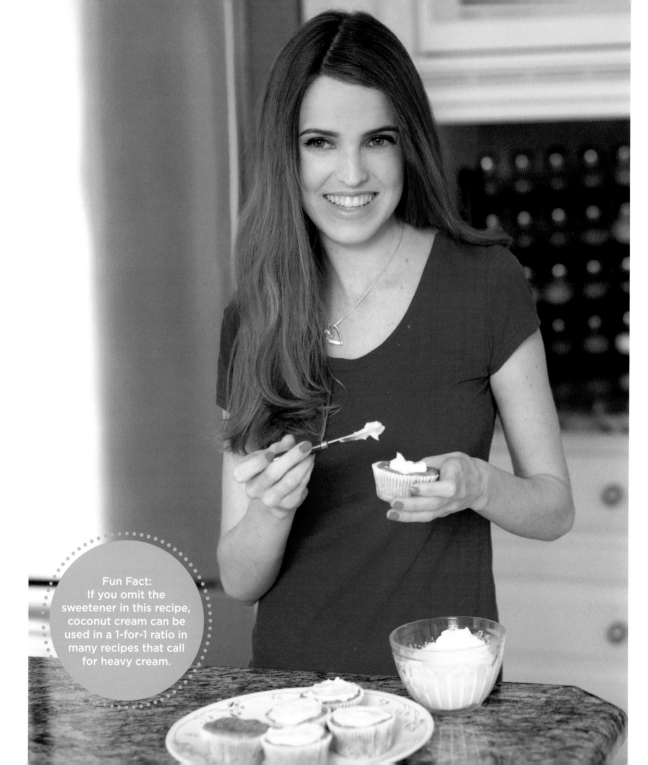

Fun Fact:
If you omit the
sweetener in this recipe,
coconut cream can be
used in a 1-for-1 ratio in
many recipes that call
for heavy cream.

coconut whipped cream

This dairy-free cream alternative can be used to top pies, cakes, ice cream sundaes, and more. It can also be used to frost cupcakes or cake. See the box on page 191 for more information about what type of coconut milk to use. makes about 1½ cups

2 (13.5-ounce) cans full-fat coconut milk (or coconut cream)	pinch pure stevia extract, or powdered sugar to taste

Refrigerate the cans of coconut milk overnight, then open the cans and transfer only the thick, creamy portion of the coconut milk into either a stand mixer or a medium mixing bowl, discarding the watery portion at the bottom of the cans. Sweeten to taste. Whip with beaters or a fork until an even, mousse-like texture is achieved.

Refrigerate leftovers in a covered container for up to 5 days. The cream gets thicker as it chills. If using this recipe as frosting, it is best to frost cupcakes or cakes just before serving due to the perishable nature of the cream.

per 1 tablespoon

Calories	30		Fat	3 grams
Fiber	0 grams		Carbs	.5 gram
Protein	.5 gram	Weight Watchers PointsPlus Value	1	

the famous cookie dough dip

Without a doubt, this is the #1 most popular recipe on chocolate coveredkatie.com. It's been featured in *Bon Appétit, Cooking Light,* and *Shape* magazines, and readers are always amazed that it really does taste just like cookie dough! Serve it as a dessert dip with graham crackers, gingersnaps, or banana slices. Or…just eat it with a spoon. (Isn't that how you're *supposed* to eat cookie dough?)

makes about 3 cups

1 (15-ounce) can chickpeas or white beans, drained and rinsed very well

$\frac{2}{3}$ cup xylitol or granulated sugar of choice

$\frac{1}{4}$ cup peanut butter or allergy-friendly alternative, or 3 tablespoons vegetable oil or melted coconut oil

3 tablespoons rolled oats, quick oats, or ground flax

2 teaspoons pure vanilla extract

$\frac{1}{8}$ heaping teaspoon baking soda

$\frac{1}{8}$ teaspoon plus $\frac{1}{16}$ teaspoon salt

up to $\frac{1}{4}$ cup milk of choice

$\frac{1}{3}$ to $\frac{1}{2}$ cup chocolate chips or homemade chocolate chips (see page 198)

In a high-quality food processor (a blender is not recommended here, but see Note), process all ingredients except milk and chocolate chips until completely smooth. Adding up to $\frac{1}{4}$ cup milk as needed, blend until the final result has the texture of cookie dough. Turn off the food processor and stir in the chocolate chips.

Refrigerate leftovers in a covered container for up to 4 days.

Note: **If you must use a blender for this recipe, do so in two batches, which gives all ingredients a chance to evenly blend. This is the only way to achieve the correct texture.**

per 1 tablespoon

Calories	25		Fat	1 gram
Fiber	.5 gram		Carbs	2.5 grams
Protein	.5 gram		Weight Watchers PointsPlus Value	1

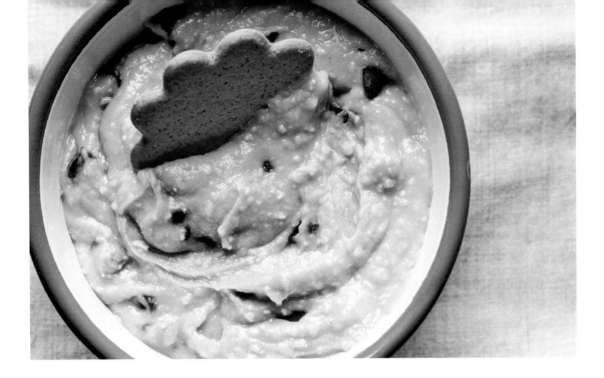

sugar-free cookie dough dip

1¼ cups pitted dates

½ cup water

1 (15-ounce) can chickpeas or white beans, drained and rinsed very well

¼ cup peanut butter, allergy-friendly substitute, or coconut or vegetable oil

2 tablespoons rolled oats

1 tablespoon plus 1 teaspoon pure vanilla extract

heaping ⅛ teaspoon baking soda

heaping ⅛ teaspoon salt

up to ¼ cup milk of choice

⅓ to ½ cup chocolate chips or homemade chocolate chips (see page 198)

In a bowl, cover the dates with the water. Let sit for 8 hours or overnight.

Transfer both the dates and their soaking liquid to a high-quality food processor (a blender is not recommended here). Add the chickpeas, peanut butter, oats, vanilla, baking soda, and salt and blend until completely smooth. Adding up to ¼ cup milk as needed, blend until the final result has the texture of cookie dough. Turn off the food processor and stir in the chocolate chips.

Refrigerate leftovers in a covered container for up to 4 days.

per 1 tablespoon

Calories	30		Fat	1 gram
Fiber	1 gram		Carbs	5.5 grams
Protein	1 gram		Weight Watchers PointsPlus Value	1

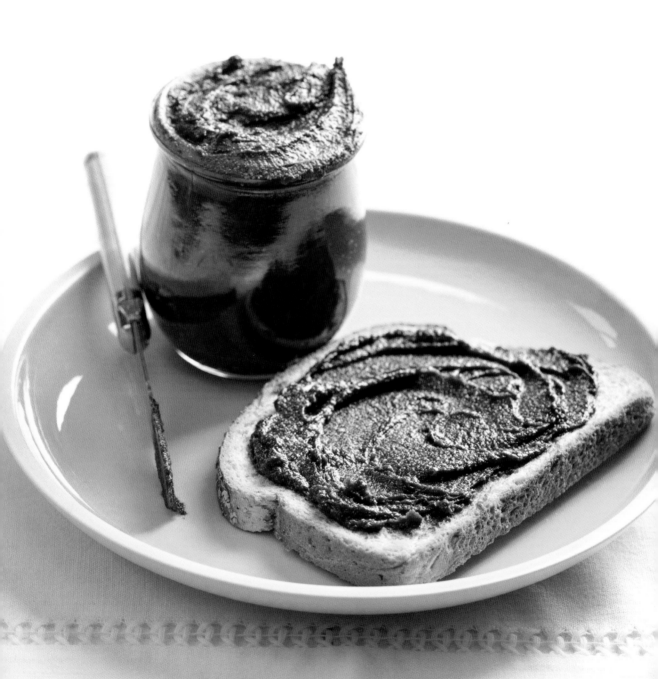

healthy chocolate notella

Store-bought Nutella is far from healthy, with 21 grams of sugar and 11 grams of fat per serving. This homemade version gives you all the deliciousness of your favorite chocolate spread with less sugar, less fat, and just half the calories. **makes about 2 cups**

2 cups raw hazelnuts

½ cup milk of choice

¼ cup cacao powder or unsweetened cocoa powder

¼ cup plus 2 tablespoons sweetener of choice (excluding stevia)

pinch pure stevia extract, or additional 1 tablespoon sweetener of choice

⅜ teaspoon salt

Preheat the oven to 400 degrees F. Roast the hazelnuts on a baking sheet for 6 to 8 minutes, until the skins darken and are toasted. Remove from the oven and allow to cool at least 10 minutes, then rub the hazelnuts together between your fingers to remove the skins. It's okay if a few stubborn skins refuse to come off.

In a high-quality food processor or Vitamix, process the nuts until a smooth and buttery texture is achieved. Add all remaining ingredients and process, stopping every so often to scrape down the sides, until the mixture achieves a smooth texture. This can take up to 6 minutes.

Use as a spread on toast or pancakes, or eat it by the spoonful. Refrigerate leftovers in a covered jar for up to 2 weeks.

per 1 tablespoon

Calories	40	Fat	3.5 grams
Fiber	1 gram	Carbs	1.5 grams
Protein	1 gram	Weight Watchers PointsPlus Value	1

healthier powdered sugar

This recipe is 100 percent sugar-free if you use xylitol, but the technique works with any granulated sugar: table sugar, Sucanat, evaporated cane juice, even coconut sugar. So the next time you run out of powdered sugar in the middle of a baking project, just make your own! makes about 1 cup

1 cup xylitol or granulated sugar of choice

1½ teaspoons arrowroot or cornstarch, optional (to prevent clumping when stored)

Whir the ingredients in a blender or Vitamix until a fine powder forms. Leftovers can be stored at room temperature in a covered container for up to 6 months.

powdered sugar glaze

To make a glaze for cookies, doughnuts, or any dessert that works well with a glaze, combine 1 cup Healthier Powdered Sugar with 1½ tablespoons milk of choice and ½ teaspoon pure vanilla extract.

Note: **Nutrition facts will be the same as those of whatever sugar you use.**

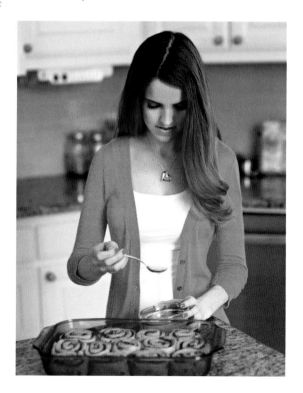

maple almond butter

With more vitamins and minerals per calorie than any other nut, almonds live up to their "superfood" status. Just one tablespoon of this sweet almond butter gives you protein, fiber, and 75 percent of your daily requirement of vitamin E. makes about 2 cups

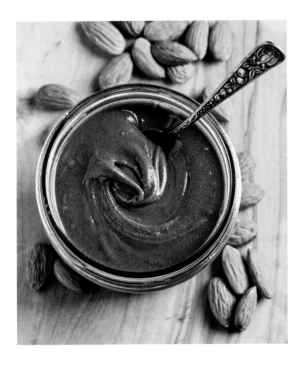

2 cups raw almonds

pinch pure stevia extract, or 2 tablespoons sweetener of choice

1 teaspoon salt

8 drops maple extract

pinch cinnamon, optional

6 tablespoons melted virgin coconut oil for a smoother texture, optional

Preheat the oven to 330 degrees F. Roast the almonds on a baking sheet for 14 minutes, or until fully toasted.

Combine all ingredients in a high-quality food processor or Vitamix and process on high, 8 to 11 minutes in a Vitamix, or 15 to 16 minutes in a food processor, scraping down the sides after each minute. The longer you blend, the smoother it will be.

Refrigerate leftovers in a covered jar for up to 1 month.

per tablespoon

Calories	70	Fat	6 grams
Fiber	2 grams	Carbs	3 grams
Protein	3 grams	Weight Watchers PointsPlus Value	2

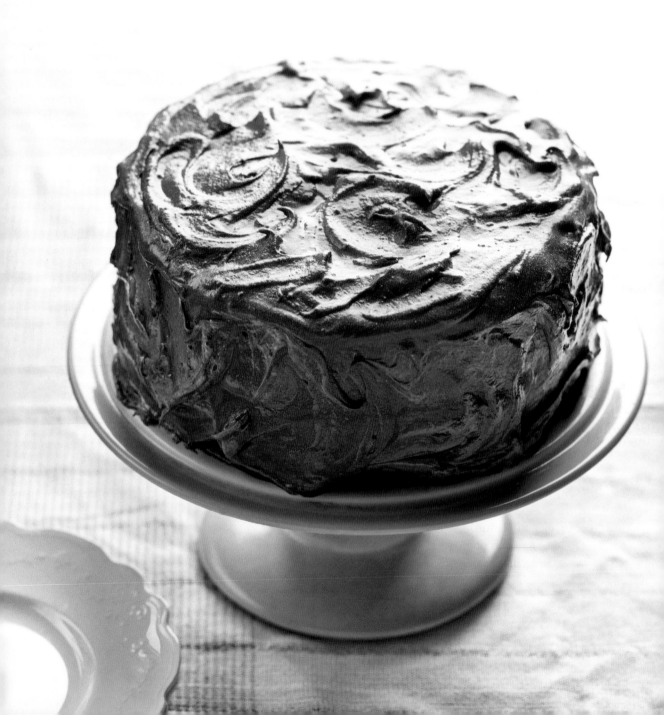

4-ingredient chocolate frosting or mousse

This frosting can be served as chocolate mousse or can be used to frost cupcakes, cakes, or even brownies.

makes enough to cover an 8-inch double layer round cake

2 (13.5-ounce) cans full-fat coconut milk (or 1 can coconut cream)

½ cup plus 2 tablespoons cacao or unsweetened cocoa powder

1 teaspoon pure vanilla extract

pinch pure stevia extract, or powdered sugar to taste

Refrigerate the cans of coconut milk overnight. Open the coconut milk and transfer only the thick, creamy portion into either a stand mixer or a medium mixing bowl, discarding the watery portion at the bottom of the cans. Add all remaining ingredients and whip with beaters or a fork until an even, mousse-like texture is achieved.

If using this as frosting, it is best to frost cupcakes or cakes just before serving due to the perishable nature of this frosting. Refrigerate leftovers in a covered container for up to 5 days. The frosting thickens as it chills.

A Note on Buying Coconut Milk

Due to the differing fat content among brands, and even within a particular brand, not all canned coconut milk will work for this recipe. A good tip is to shake the can while at the store. If you can hear the milk splashing around, put the can back and look for one that sounds more solid. I have had good luck with Thai Kitchen Organic. Or, for a foolproof solution, use coconut cream, which can be found at Trader Joe's and at Asian grocery stores. Do not use the coconut milk that comes in a carton for this recipe; it is not the same as canned coconut milk.

per tablespoon

Calories	30		Fat	3.5 grams
Fiber	1 gram		Carbs	1.5 grams
Protein	.5 gram	Weight Watchers PointsPlus Value	1	

healthier cream cheese frosting

This frosting is good on basically anything: cinnamon rolls, cupcakes, cake, and even pancakes. It's especially good if you spread it on slices of Chocolate Chip Pumpkin Bread (page 84). **makes about 1¼ cups**

1½ cups cream cheese spread (such as Tofutti's non-hydrogenated Better Than Cream Cheese or Daiya's cream cheese–style spread)

1 cup mashed firm silken tofu (I recommend Mori-Nu)*

2 teaspoons pure vanilla extract

pinch pure stevia extract, or 3 to 5 tablespoons powdered sugar

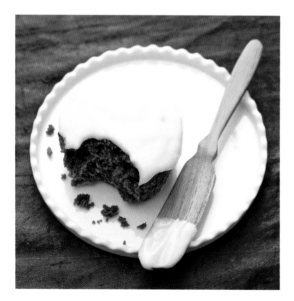

Blend all ingredients together in a food processor, blender, or Vitamix until completely smooth.

Taste, then add additional sweetener if needed. If using this recipe to top cupcakes or cake, frost just before serving due to the perishable nature of the ingredients. Refrigerate leftovers in a covered container for 3 to 4 days.

per tablespoon

Calories	20	Fat	1.5 grams
Fiber	0 grams	Carbs	.5 gram
Protein	.5 gram	Weight Watchers PointsPlus Value	0

*For a soy-free frosting, replace the tofu with 1 cup additional cream cheese spread.

strawberry cupcake frosting

Lusciously thick, without any of the chemicals, shortening, or corn syrup found in store-bought frostings. The berries turn this frosting a brilliant shade of pink—no food coloring required! **makes about 1 cup**

1 (13.5-ounce) can full-fat coconut milk* (or 1 can coconut cream)

2 strawberries, stems cut off

1/4 teaspoon pure vanilla extract

1/16 teaspoon pure stevia, or 2 tablespoons powdered sugar

tiny pinch salt

Refrigerate the cans of coconut milk overnight. Open the coconut milk and transfer only the thick, creamy portion to a blender. Add the berries, vanilla extract, sweetener, and salt and blend until a mousse-like texture is achieved.

If using this as frosting, it is best to frost cupcakes or cakes just before serving due to the perishable nature of this frosting. Refrigerate leftovers in a covered container for up to 5 days. The frosting thickens as it chills.

per tablespoon

Calories	30	Fat	3 grams
Fiber	0 grams	Carbs	0.5 gram
Protein	.5 gram	Weight Watchers PointsPlus Value	1

*See the box on page 191 for more information about what type of coconut milk to use.

chocolate cookie pie crust

Completely free of lard, preservatives, and flour, this is a much healthier alternative to store-bought pie crust and will work with many different types of pie fillings. Try it as a base for either the Chocolate Infinity Pie (page 146) or the Red Velvet Fudge Pie (page 154).

makes one 8½-inch pie crust (10 servings)

1 cup pitted dates

1 cup almonds

⅓ cup walnuts

⅓ cup cacao powder or unsweetened cocoa powder

1 tablespoon water

¼ teaspoon salt

per serving

Calories	130	Fat	7 grams
Fiber	4 grams	Carbs	15 grams
Protein	4 grams	Weight Watchers PointsPlus Value	3

Line the bottom of an 8½-inch springform pan with parchment paper.

Combine all ingredients in a high-quality food processor and process until fine crumbs form. Press the dough into the prepared pan, pressing up the sides. Freeze at least 4 hours, until set. If desired, this recipe can be made ahead of time. Cover the pan and store in the freezer for up to 2 weeks.

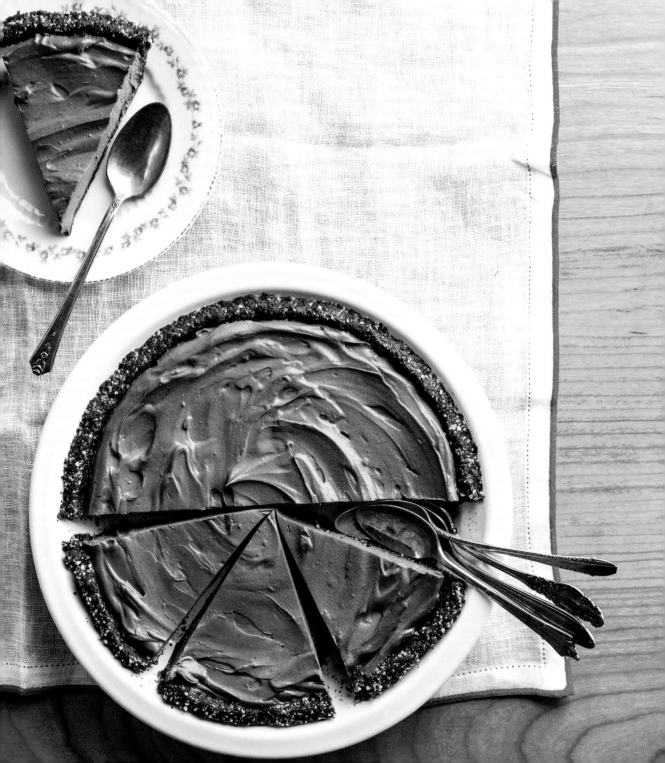

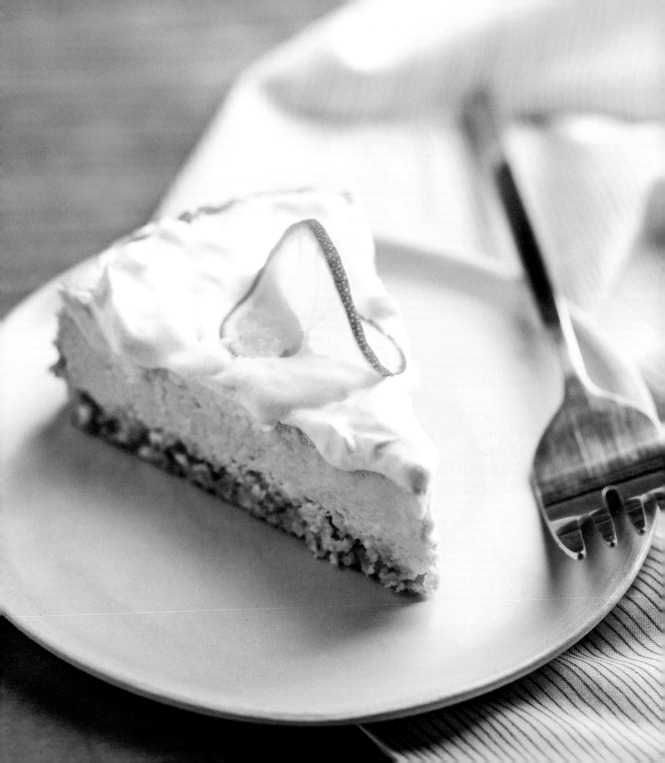

oatmeal cookie pie crust

Rolled oats make up the bulk of this pie crust, which helps to keep the fat down, increases the fiber, and eliminates the need for any flour whatsoever. It's the perfect base for the Key Lime Pie Cheesecake (page 157). **makes one 8½-inch pie crust (10 servings)**

1 cup rolled oats

½ cup shredded coconut

¼ cup vegetable oil or melted coconut oil

pinch pure stevia extract, or 1 tablespoon granulated sugar of choice

¼ teaspoon salt

per serving

Calories	90	Fat	7 grams
Fiber	2 grams	Carbs	6 grams
Protein	2 grams	Weight Watchers PointsPlus Value	2

Line the bottom of an 8½-inch springform pan with parchment paper.

Combine all ingredients in a high-quality food processor and process until fine crumbs form. Press the dough into the prepared pan, pressing up the sides. If desired, the pie crust can be made ahead of time. Cover the pan and store in the freezer for up to 2 weeks.

make your own chocolate chips!

Let your creativity go absolutely crazy with this customizable homemade chocolate chip recipe. Add a pinch of cinnamon or a few drops of peppermint or almond extract, or keep it simple with classic dark chocolate. The only problem with these chips is that I eat them so quickly that by the time I get around to making a recipe in which to use them, there are rarely ever any left! **makes about ½ cup**

¼ **cup virgin coconut oil, melted**

1 tablespoon pure maple syrup or liquid sweetener of choice

¼ **cup cacao powder or unsweetened cocoa powder**

extracts or add-ins of choice, optional

In a medium bowl, combine the coconut oil and maple syrup. Add the cacao powder and stir until a thick sauce forms. If necessary, add more coconut oil for a thinner consistency.

Transfer to a resealable plastic bag and smush into a bar shape, or pour into candy molds or a flat container. Freeze until solid, at least 2 hours.

Remove from the freezer and break into pieces, using a knife or your hands. Store in the freezer for up to 3 months. These chips work wonderfully when added to raw treats (such as the I ♥ Chocolate Chip Cookie Dough Bars, page 49). However, they melt when heated and therefore will not hold their shape in baked cookies.

per tablespoon

Calories	70	Fat	1 gram
Fiber	7 grams	Carbs	3 grams
Protein	.5 gram	Weight Watchers PointsPlus Value	2

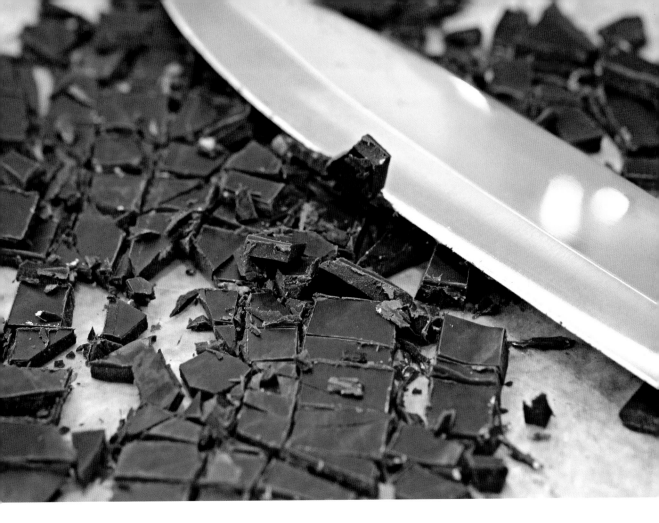

sugar-free chocolate chips

makes about ½ cup

....

½ cup plus 1 tablespoon cacao powder or unsweetened cocoa powder

¼ cup melted virgin coconut oil, plus more if needed

20 drops NuNaturals alcohol-free vanilla stevia, plus more to taste

extra coconut oil for a thinner consistency, if needed

extracts or add-ins of choice, optional

Follow the directions and storage instructions on the opposite page.

per tablespoon

Calories	70	Fat	1 gram
Fiber	7 grams	Carbs	3 grams
Protein	2 grams	Weight Watchers PointsPlus Value	2

stevia conversion chart

The amount of stevia to use in a recipe will depend greatly on the brand of stevia. Recipes in this book call for concentrated stevia extract in its pure form, which has not been cut with other ingredients such as maltodextrin, dextrose, or erythritol.

The following chart pertains only to NuNaturals stevia, which is the only brand I've found to not have an unpleasant aftertaste when used in small amounts in recipes.

pinch pure stevia extract ($1/_{32}$ teaspoon)	1 tablespoon sugar
$1/_{16}$ teaspoon pure stevia extract	2 tablespoons sugar
1 NuNaturals stevia packet	1 tablespoon sugar
1 NuNaturals stevia packet	$1/_2$ teaspoon NuNaturals powder
1 NuNaturals stevia packet	$1/_{32}$ teaspoon pure stevia extract
1 packet NuNaturals No Carbs Blend	1 tablespoon sugar
7 drops Alcohol Free Vanilla Stevia (liquid)	2 teaspoons sugar

When a recipe calls for pure stevia extract, feel free to substitute NuNaturals packets or powder in accordance with the chart above. However, when a recipe does not specifically mention "stevia" or "sweetener of choice" as an option, do not try to substitute stevia, as doing so may negatively alter the texture and taste of a recipe.

metric conversion charts

Use these charts as a guideline. In the United States, recipe ingredient lists are usually based on volume rather than weight. Baking recipes (breads, muffins, cakes) do require precision, so exact conversions are necessary.

u.s. to metric conversion, flour

U.S.	Metric
¼ cup	30 grams
½ cup	60 grams
¾ cup	90 grams
1 cup	120 grams

u.s. to metric conversion, temperature

Degrees Fahrenheit	Degrees Celsius
325	163
350	177
375	191
400	204
425	218
450	232
475	246

u.s. to metric conversion, volume, liquid

U.S.	Metric
¼ teaspoon	1 milliliter
½ teaspoon	2 milliliters
1 teaspoon	5 milliliters
1 fluid ounce (2 tablespoons)	30 milliliters
2 fluid ounces (¼ cup)	60 milliliters
8 fluid ounces (1 cup)	240 milliliters
16 fluid ounces (1 pint)	480 milliliters
32 fluid ounces (1 quart)	950 milliliters (.95 liter)
128 fluid ounces (1 gallon)	3.75 liters

index

agave, raw, about, 16
all-purpose flour, about, 17
almond butter
    about, 18
    Maple Almond Butter, 189
    in Pumpkin Pie Granola Bars, 45
    Real-Food Protein Bars, 53
almonds
    in Chocolate Cookie Pie Crust,
        194
    in Midnight Chocolate Crunch
        Granola, 80
    in Pumpkin Pie Granola Bars, 45
altitude considerations, 20
American as Apple Pie Muffins, 100
Anytime Chocolate Fudge Balls, 58
apples
    American as Apple Pie Muffins,
        100
    in The "No More Hunger"
        Breakfast Bowl, 75
avocados
    in The Chocolate Mudslide, 130
    selection tip, 131

Baked Peaches with Yogurt
        and Granola, 87
baking pans, 15
baking sheets, 15
Bananaccino, The, 128
bananas
    freezer storage tip, 106
    The Bananaccino, 128
    Chai Banana Soft Serve, 109
    Chocolate Banana Bread
        Cupcakes, 165
    in Coconut Frosting, 50
    in Elvis Peanut Butter Pancakes,
        72
    in Mint Chocolate Chip
        Milkshake, 124
    in Real-Food Protein Bars, 53

    in Peanut Butter Pudding Pops,
        116
    in Superfood Chocolate Bowls,
        76
barley, in The "No More Hunger"
        Breakfast Bowl, 75
bars
    Carrot Cake Bars with Coconut
        Frosting, 50
    Chocolate Raspberry Crumble
        Bars, 46
    I ♥ Chocolate Chip Cookie
        Dough Bars, 49
    Pumpkin Pie Granola
        Bars, 45
    Real-Food Protein Bars, 53
beans
    in Deep Dish Cookie Pie, 138
    in Double Chocolate
        Peppermint Brownies, 40
    in The Famous Cookie Dough
        Dip, 184
    in Peanut Butter Fudge
        Brownie Dip, 176
berries. See blueberries;
        raspberries; strawberries
Berry Oatmeal Crumble, 153
blenders
    magic bullet, 14
    Vitamix, 14
blueberries
    Berry Oatmeal Crumble, 153
    The Blueberry Beauty Queen,
        123
    Blueberry Morning Baked
        Oatmeal, 68
    Blueberry Silk Pie, 161
Blueberry Beauty Queen,
        The, 123
Blueberry Morning Baked
        Oatmeal, 68
Blueberry Silk Pie, 161

Bob's Red Mill gluten-free all-
        purpose baking flour,
        about, 17
bran flakes. See flake cereals
breads
    Chocolate Banana Bread
        Cupcakes, 165
    Chocolate Chip Pumpkin Bread,
        84
breakfast desserts
    American as Apple Pie Muffins,
        100
    Baked Peaches with Yogurt and
        Granola, 87
    Blueberry Morning Baked
        Oatmeal, 68
    Cappuccino Chocolate Chip
        Mini Muffins, 99
    Chocoholic Glazed Doughnuts,
        88
    Chocolate Brownie Waffles, 64
    Chocolate Chip Pumpkin Bread,
        84
    Cinnamon Raisin Granola, 79
    The Creamiest Oatmeal of Your
        Life, 83
    Elvis Peanut Butter Pancakes,
        72
    Frosted Lemon Doughnuts, 91
    Gluten-Free Chocolate Chip
        Pancakes, 71
    Ironman Muffins, 95
    Midnight Chocolate Crunch
        Granola, 80
    The "No More Hunger"
        Breakfast Bowl, 75
    Pumpkin Breakfast Pudding, 67
    Raspberry Orange Corn
        Muffins, 96
    Sunday Morning Cinnamon
        Rolls, 92
    Superfood Chocolate Bowls, 76

brownies
    Chocolate Brownie Waffles, 64
    Double Chocolate Peppermint
        Brownies, 40
    Peanut Butter Fudge Brownie
        Dip, 176
    Secretly Healthy Brownies, 38
    The Ultimate Unbaked
        Brownies, 42

cakes. See also cupcakes
    Chocolate Birthday Cake Pops,
        170
    Chocolate Obsession Cake, 142
    Key Lime Pie Cheesecake, 157
    New York–Style Cheesecake, 141
    Pink Princess Cake, 145
Cappuccino Chocolate Chip Mini
    Muffins, 99
Carrot Cake Bars with Coconut
    Frosting, 50
Carrot Raisin Cookie Bites, 57
carrots
    Carrot Cake Bars with Coconut
        Frosting, 50
    Carrot Raisin Cookie Bites, 57
    in The Creamiest Oatmeal of
        Your Life, 83
Cashew Cream Mini Tarts, 149
cashews
    Cashew Cream Mini Tarts, 149
    in Coffee Chocolate Chip Ice
        Cream, 104
    in Lemon Meltaway Pie, 162
    in Peppermint White Hot
        Chocolate, 132
cauliflower, in Lemon Meltaway
    Pie, 162
cereal flakes. See flake cereals
Chai Banana Soft Serve, 109
cheesecakes
    Key Lime Pie Cheesecake, 157
    New York–Style Cheesecake, 141
cherries
    Cherry Peach Crumble Tart, 150
    The Chocolate-Covered Cherry,
        127

Cherry Peach Crumble Tart, 150
Chewy Oatmeal Crinkle Cookies,
    29
Chia Power Pudding, Chocolate,
    180
Chocoholic Glazed Doughnuts,
    88
chocolate. See also chocolate
    chips
  about, 19
  benefits of, 11
  melting tip, 21
  breakfast desserts
    Cappuccino Chocolate Chip
        Mini Muffins, 99
    Chocoholic Glazed
        Doughnuts, 88
    Chocolate Brownie Waffles, 64
    Midnight Chocolate Crunch
        Granola, 80
    Superfood Chocolate Bowls, 76
  cookies, brownies and bars
    Anytime Chocolate Fudge
        Balls, 58
    Chocolate-Covered Thin
        Mintz, 34
    Chocolate Peanut Butter
        Buckeyes, 54
    Chocolate Pixie Cookies, 25
    Chocolate Raspberry
        Crumble Bars, 46
    Double Chocolate
        Peppermint Brownies, 40
    I ♥ Chocolate Chip Cookie
        Dough Bars, 49
    Secretly Healthy Brownies, 38
    The Ultimate Unbaked
        Brownies, 42
  drinks
    The Chocolate-Covered
        Cherry, 127
    The Chocolate Mudslide, 130
    Frozen Hot Chocolate, 120
    The Mint Chocolate Chip
        Milkshake, 124
    Peppermint White Hot
        Chocolate, 133

ice cream
    Chocolate Peanut Butter Cup
        Ice Cream, 112
    Coffee Chocolate Chip Ice
        Cream, 104
pies, cakes and cupcakes
    Chocolate Banana Bread
        Cupcakes, 165
    Chocolate Birthday Cake
        Pops, 170
    Chocolate Cookie Pie Crust,
        194
    Chocolate Infinity Pie, 146
    Chocolate Obsession Cake,
        142
    Chocolate Zucchini
        Cupcakes, 169
    Red Velvet Fudge Pie, 154
puddings, dips and more
    Chocolate Chia Power
        Pudding, 180
    4-Ingredient Chocolate
        Frosting or Mousse, 191
    Healthy Chocolate Notella, 187
    Peanut Butter Fudge Brownie
        Dip, 176
Chocolate Banana Bread
    Cupcakes, 165
Chocolate Birthday Cake Pops,
    170
Chocolate Brownie Waffles, 64
Chocolate Chia Power Pudding,
    180
Chocolate Chip Pumpkin Bread, 84
chocolate chips
    Cappuccino Chocolate Chip
        Mini Muffins, 99
    Chocolate Chip Pumpkin Bread,
        84
    Chocolate Infinity Pie, 146
    Chocolate Obsession Cake, 142
    Coffee Chocolate Chip Ice
        Cream, 104
    Flourless Chocolate Chip
        Cookies, 30
    Gluten-Free Chocolate Chip
        Pancakes, 71

chocolate chips (*cont.*)

I ♥ Chocolate Chip Cookie Dough Bars, 49

Make Your Own Chocolate Chips!, 198

Mint Chocolate Chip Milkshake, 124

Sugar-Free Chocolate Chips, 199

Chocolate Cookie Pie Crust, 194

Chocolate-Covered Cherry, The, 127

Chocolate-Covered Katie (blog), 10

Chocolate-Covered Thin Mintz, 34

Chocolate Infinity Pie, 146

Chocolate Mudslide, The, 130

Chocolate Obsession Cake, 142

Chocolate Peanut Butter Buckeyes, 54

Chocolate Peanut Butter Cup Ice Cream, 112

Chocolate Pixie Cookies, 25

Chocolate Raspberry Crumble Bars, 46

Chocolate Zucchini Cupcakes, 169

cholesterol, 12, 17–18

Cinnamon Raisin Granola, 79

Cinnamon Rolls, Sunday Morning, 92

Classic Rice Pudding, 179

climate considerations, 20

coconut butter, about, 18

Coconut Cloud Cupcakes, 166

coconut flour, about, 16–17

coconut milk

about canned, 19

buying tip, 191

in Coconut Whipped Cream, 183

in 4-Ingredient Chocolate Frosting or Mousse, 191

in Frozen Hot Chocolate, 120

in Pure Bliss Vanilla Ice Cream, 107

in Strawberry Shortcakes, 173

coconut oil, virgin

about, 18–19

melted, mixing ingredients, 20

coconut sugar, 15–16

Coconut Whipped Cream, 183

coffee

in The Bananaccino, 128

Cappuccino Chocolate Chip Mini Muffins, 99

Coffee Chocolate Chip Ice Cream, 104

Coffee Chocolate Chip Ice Cream, 104

cookies

storage tip, 24

Anytime Chocolate Fudge Balls, 58

Carrot Raisin Cookie Bites, 57

Chewy Oatmeal Crinkle Cookies, 29

Chocolate-Covered Thin Mintz, 34

Chocolate Peanut Butter Buckeyes, 54

Chocolate Pixie Cookies, 25

Deep Dish Cookie Pie, 138

The Famous Cookie Dough Dip, 184

Flourless Chocolate Chip Cookies, 30

Gingerbread Molasses Cookies, 33

Oatmeal Raisin Cookies, 31

Sinless Peanut Butter Cookies, 26

Special CCK No-Bake Cookies, 37

cooking terms, 19

cooking tips, 19–21

Corn Muffins, Raspberry Orange, 96

cravings, 10

Cream Cheese Frosting, Healthier, 192

Creamiest Oatmeal of Your Life, The, 83

crumbles

Berry Oatmeal Crumble, 153

Cherry Peach Crumble Tart, 150

Chocolate Raspberry Crumble Bars, 46

cupcake liners, 15

cupcakes

Chocolate Banana Bread Cupcakes, 165

Chocolate Zucchini Cupcakes, 169

Coconut Cloud Cupcakes, 166

Strawberry Cupcake Frosting, 193

Dairy-Free Milk, Homemade, 134

dark chocolate, benefits of eating, 11

dates

about, 16

in Anytime Chocolate Fudge Balls, 58

in Chocolate Cookie Pie Crust, 194

in I ♥ Chocolate Chip Cookie Dough Bars, 49

in The Ultimate Unbaked Brownies, 42

Deep Dish Cookie Pie, 138

Sugar-Free, 139

diet books, 10

dips

The Famous Cookie Dough Dip, 184

Peanut Butter Fudge Brownie Dip, 176

Sugar-Free Cookie Dough Dip, 185

double boiler method, for melting chocolate, 21

Double Chocolate Peppermint Brownies, 40

doughnuts

Chocoholic Glazed Doughnuts, 88

Frosted Lemon Doughnuts, 91

Elvis Peanut Butter Pancakes, 72

Famous Cookie Dough Dip, The, 184

fats, 17–19

flake cereals
    in Ironman Muffins, 95
    in Pumpkin Breakfast Pudding, 67
    in Special CCK No-Bake Cookies, 36
flavonols, in dark chocolate, 11
flaxmeal (ground flax), about, 18
Flourless Chocolate Chip Cookies, 30
flours, 16–17
food processor, 14
food scale, 15
4-Ingredient Chocolate Frosting or Mousse, 191
Frosted Lemon Doughnuts, 91
frostings
    4-Ingredient Chocolate Frosting or Mousse, 191
    Healthier Cream Cheese Frosting, 192
    Strawberry Cupcake Frosting, 193
Frozen Hot Chocolate, 120
fudge
    Anytime Chocolate Fudge Balls, 58
    Peanut Butter Fudge Brownie Dip, 176
    Red Velvet Fudge Pie, 155

Gingerbread Molasses Cookies, 33
gluten-free all-purpose baking flour, Bob's Red Mill, about, 17
gluten-free options
    American as Apple Pie Muffins, 100
    Cappuccino Chocolate Chip Mini Muffins, 99
    Carrot Cake Bars with Coconut Frosting, 50
    Cherry Peach Crumble Tart, 151
    Chewy Oatmeal Crinkle Cookies, 29
    Chocoholic Glazed Doughnuts, 88

Chocolate Banana Bread Cupcakes, 165
Chocolate Chip Pancakes, 71
Chocolate Chip Pumpkin Bread, 84
Chocolate Obsession Cake, 142
Chocolate Pixie Cookies, 25
Chocolate Raspberry Crumble Bars, 47
Chocolate Zucchini Cupcakes, 169
Coconut Cloud Cupcakes, 166
Frosted Lemon Doughnuts, 91
Gingerbread Molasses Cookies, 33
Ironman Muffins, 95
Pink Princess Cake, 145
Raspberry Orange Corn Muffins, 96
Strawberry Shortcakes, 173
granola
    Baked Peaches with Yogurt and Granola, 87
    Cinnamon Raisin Granola, 79
    Midnight Chocolate Crunch Granola, 80
    Pumpkin Pie Granola Bars, 45
ground flax (flaxmeal), about, 18

hazelnuts
    in Healthy Chocolate Notella, 187
    in Homemade Dairy-Free Milk, 134
Healthier Cream Cheese Frosting, 192
Healthier Powdered Sugar, 188
Healthy Brownies, Secretly, 38
Healthy Chocolate Notella, 187
Homemade Dairy-Free Milk, 134
Hot Chocolate
    Frozen, 118
    Peppermint White, 133

ice cream
    freezing methods, 104–5
    storage tip, 105
    Chai Banana Soft Serve, 109

Chocolate Peanut Butter Cup Ice Cream, 112
Coffee Chocolate Chip Ice Cream, 104
Frozen Hot Chocolate, 120
Peanut Butter Pudding Pops, 116
Pistachio Ice Cream, 110
Pure Bliss Vanilla Ice Cream, 106
Sunrise Mango Sherbet, 115
I ♥ Chocolate Chip Cookie Dough Bars, 49
ingredients list, 15–19
    fats, 17–19
    flours, 16–17
    sweeteners, 15–16
Ironman Muffins, 95

Key Lime Pie Cheesecake, 157
kitchen tools, 14–15

lemon
    Frosted Lemon Doughnuts, 91
    Lemon Meltaway Pie, 162
Lime Pie Cheesecake, Key, 157

macadamia nuts
    in Blueberry Silk Pie, 161
    in Coffee Chocolate Chip Ice Cream, 104
    in Homemade Dairy-Free Milk, 134
    in Lemon Meltaway Pie, 162
magic bullet blenders, 14
Make Your Own Chocolate Chips!, 198
Mango Sherbet, Sunrise, 115
Maple Almond Butter, 189
measuring spoons, 14–15
melting chocolate, 21
metric conversion chart, 201
microwave method, for melting chocolate, 21
Midnight Chocolate Crunch Granola, 80
milkshakes
    The Chocolate Mudslide, 130
    The Mint Chocolate Chip Milkshake, 124

Mint Chocolate Chip Milkshake, 124

Miss Scarlet Strawberry Pie, 158

mixing bowls, 15

molasses (blackstrap)
about, 15
Gingerbread Molasses Cookies, 33

Mousse, 4-Ingredient Chocolate Frosting or, 191

muffins
American as Apple Pie Muffins, 100
Cappuccino Chocolate Chip Mini Muffins, 99
Ironman Muffins, 95
Raspberry Orange Corn Muffins, 96

New York–Style Cheesecake, 141

no-bake (unbake) cookies, bars, brownies
Anytime Chocolate Fudge Balls, 58
Carrot Raisin Cookie Bites, 57
I ♥ Chocolate Chip Cookie Dough Bars, 49
Peanut Butter & Jelly Candy Cups, 60
Real-Food Protein Bars, 53
Special CCK No-Bake Cookies, 36
The Ultimate Unbaked Brownies, 42

"No More Hunger" Breakfast Bowl, The, 75

Notella, Healthy Chocolate, 187

nut butters, 18. See also specific nut butters

nuts. See also specific nuts
in Homemade Dairy-Free Milk, 134

oat flour
about, 17
in Gingerbread Molasses Cookies, 33

Oatmeal Cookie Pie Crust, 197

Oatmeal Raisin Cookies, 31

oats (oatmeal)
Berry Oatmeal Crumble, 153
Blueberry Morning Baked Oatmeal, 68
Chewy Oatmeal Crinkle Cookies, 29
in Cinnamon Raisin Granola, 79
The Creamiest Oatmeal of Your Life, 83
in Deep Dish Cookie Pie, 138
Flourless Chocolate Chip Cookies, 30
in Midnight Chocolate Crunch Granola, 80
Oatmeal Cookie Pie Crust, 197
Oatmeal Raisin Cookies, 31
in Pumpkin Pie Granola Bars, 45

oven calibration, 20

pancakes
Elvis Peanut Butter Pancakes, 72
Gluten-Free Chocolate Chip Pancakes, 71

parchment paper, 15

pastry flour, whole wheat, about, 17

peaches
Baked Peaches with Yogurt and Granola, 87
Cherry Peach Crumble Tart, 150
The Passionate Peach, 132

peanut butter
about, 18
Chocolate Peanut Butter Buckeyes, 54
Chocolate Peanut Butter Cup Ice Cream, 112
Elvis Peanut Butter Pancakes, 72
in The Famous Cookie Dough Dip, 184
Peanut Butter Fudge Brownie Dip, 176
Peanut Butter & Jelly Candy Cups, 60
Peanut Butter Pudding Pops, 116

powdered. See powdered peanut butter
Sinless Peanut Butter Cookies, 26
in Special CCK No-Bake Cookies, 37
Peanut Butter Fudge Brownie Dip, 176
Peanut Butter & Jelly Candy Cups, 60
Peanut Butter Pudding Pops, 116

pecans, in Anytime Chocolate Fudge Balls, 58

peppermint
in Chocolate-Covered Thin Mintz, 34
Double Chocolate Peppermint Brownies, 40
Peppermint White Hot Chocolate, 133

Peppermint White Hot Chocolate, 133

pie crusts
Chocolate Cookie Pie Crust, 194
Oatmeal Cookie Pie Crust, 197

pies
Blueberry Silk Pie, 161
Chocolate Infinity Pie, 146
Deep Dish Cookie Pie, 138
Lemon Meltaway Pie, 162
Miss Scarlet Strawberry Pie, 158
Red Velvet Fudge Pie, 154

pineapple
in Coconut Cloud Cupcakes, 166
Tropical Pineapple Popsicles, 119

Pink Princess Cake, 145

Pistachio Ice Cream, 110

popsicles/pops
Chocolate Birthday Cake Pops, 170
Peanut Butter Pudding Pops, 116
Tropical Pineapple Popsicles, 119

powdered peanut butter, 59
Peanut Butter & Jelly Candy Cups, 60

Powdered Sugar, Healthier, 188

Powdered Sugar Glaze, 188

Protein Bars, Real-Food, 53
puddings
    Chocolate Chia Power Pudding,
        180
    Classic Rice Pudding, 179
    Peanut Butter Pudding Pops,
        116
    Pumpkin Breakfast Pudding, 67
pumpkin
    Chocolate Chip Pumpkin Bread,
        84
    Pumpkin Breakfast Pudding, 67
    Pumpkin Pie Granola Bars, 45
Pumpkin Breakfast Pudding, 67
Pumpkin Pie Granola Bars, 45
Pure Bliss Vanilla Ice Cream, 106

quinoa, in Superfood Chocolate
        Bowls, 76

raisins
    Carrot Raisin Cookie Bites, 57
    Cinnamon Raisin Granola, 79
    in Classic Rice Pudding, 179
    Oatmeal Raisin Cookies, 31
raspberries
    in Berry Oatmeal Crumble, 153
    Chocolate Raspberry Crumble
        Bars, 46
    in Midnight Chocolate Crunch
        Granola, 80
    Raspberry Orange Corn
        Muffins, 96
    in Red Velvet Fudge Pie, 154
Raspberry Orange Corn Muffins,
    96
raw agave, about, 16
Real-Food Protein Bars, 53
recipe substitutions, 19–20
Red Velvet Fudge Pie, 154
Rice Pudding, Classic, 179

Secretly Healthy Brownies, 38
Sherbet, Sunrise Mango, 115
Shortcakes, Strawberry, 173
Sinless Peanut Butter Cookies, 26
smoothies

The Bananaccino, 128
The Blueberry Beauty Queen,
    123
The Chocolate-Covered Cherry,
    127
The Mint Chocolate Chip
    Milkshake, 124
The Passionate Peach, 132
sorghum flour
    about, 68
    in Gluten-Free Chocolate Chip
        Pancakes, 71
Special CCK No-Bake Cookies, 37
spelt flour, whole grain, about, 17
spinach
    in The Chocolate-Covered
        Cherry, 127
    in The Mint Chocolate Chip
        Milkshake, 124
spreads, Healthy Chocolate
    Notella, 187
stevia
    about, 16
    conversion chart, 200
strawberries
    Miss Scarlet Strawberry Pie,
        158
    in The Passionate Peach, 132
    in Pink Princess Cake, 145
    Strawberry Cupcake Frosting,
        193
    Strawberry Shortcakes, 173
Strawberry Cupcake Frosting, 193
Strawberry Shortcakes, 173
Sucanat, about, 16
Sugar-Free Chocolate Chips, 199
Sugar-Free Cookie Dough Dip,
    185
Sugar-Free Deep Dish Cookie
    Pie, 139
Sunday Morning Cinnamon Rolls,
    92
Sunrise Mango Sherbet, 115
Superfood Chocolate Bowls, 76
sweeteners, 15–16. See also
    specific sweeteners
sweets cravings, 10

tarts
    Cashew Cream Mini Tarts, 149
    Cherry Peach Crumble Tart, 150
Thin Mintz, Chocolate-Covered,
    34
tofu
    in Chocolate Infinity Pie, 146
    in Healthier Cream Cheese
        Frosting, 192
    in Key Lime Pie Cheesecake,
        157
    in New York–Style Cheesecake,
        141
    in Peppermint White Hot
        Chocolate, 133
tools, 14–15
Tropical Pineapple Popsicles, 119
troubleshooting tips, 19–21

Ultimate Unbaked Brownies,
        The, 42

Vanilla Ice Cream, Pure Bliss, 106
virgin coconut oil
    about, 18–19
    melted, mixing ingredients, 20
Vitamix blenders, 14

Waffles, Chocolate Brownie, 64
walnuts
    Cashew Cream Mini Tarts, 149
    in Chocolate Cookie Pie Crust,
        194
    in The Ultimate Unbaked
        Brownies, 42
water bath, for melting chocolate,
    21
Whipped Cream, Coconut, 183
whole grain spelt flour, about, 17
whole wheat pastry flour, about, 17

xylitol, about, 16

Yogurt and Granola, Baked
        Peaches with, 87

Zucchini Chocolate Cupcakes, 169

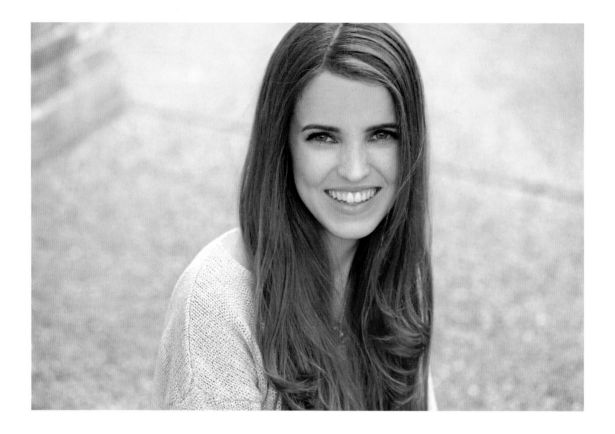

about the author

Katie Higgins is a writer, recipe developer, and photographer who runs *Chocolate-Covered Katie*, an award-winning food blog with over six million visitors every month. She is passionate about creating healthier versions of traditional decadent treats, proving one needn't give up eating dessert to be healthy.

Katie's work has been featured by media outlets such as CNN, ABC, *Time, Glamour,* the Food Network, and the *Huffington Post,* and her website won the Foodbuzz Best Baking Blog Award of 2011.

Katie grew up in England, Japan, Philadelphia, the Philippines, China, and Texas, and she currently resides in the Washington, DC, area with two crazy rescue dogs and a kitchen cabinet full of chocolate. Her blog can be found at chocolatecoveredkatie.com.